Steamy

Steamy

A MENOPAUSE SYMPTOMOLOGY

SUSAN HOLBROOK

COACH HOUSE BOOKS, TORONTO

first edition

Published with the generous assistance of the Canada Council for the Arts and the Ontario Arts Council. Coach House Books also acknowledges the support of the Government of Canada through the Canada Book Fund and the Government of Ontario through the Ontario Book Publishing Tax Credit.

LIBRARY AND ARCHIVES CANADA CATALOGUING IN PUBLICATION

Title: Steamy : a menopause symptomology / by Susan Holbrook.
Names: Holbrook, Susan, 1967- author
Identifiers: Canadiana (print) 20250113929 | Canadiana (ebook) 20250135108 | ISBN 9781552455029 (softcover) | ISBN 9781770568440 (EPUB) | ISBN 9781770568563 (PDF)
Subjects: LCSH: Holbrook, Susan, 1967-—Health. | LCSH: Menopause—Humor. | LCGFT: Autobiographies. | LCGFT: Humor.
Classification: LCC RG186 .H65 2025 | DDC 612.6/65—dc23

Steamy: A Menopause Symptomology is available as an ebook: ISBN 978 1 77056 844 0 (EPUB), ISBN 978 1 77056 856 3 (PDF)

Purchase of the print version of this book entitles you to a free digital copy. To claim your ebook of this title, please email sales@chbooks.com with proof of purchase. (Coach House Books reserves the right to terminate the free digital download offer at any time.)

for all the hotties

'When describing this book to others, I initially felt a mixture of defiance and defensiveness; I was embarrassed by the subject and would blush, then feel intensely irritated. There was usually a polite suppressed spasm of alarm, a fleeting look of distaste, and often genuine surprise, if not shock, at the very thought.'

– Louise Foxcroft, Hot Flushes, Cold Science:
A History of the Modern Menopause

'And they're like, "Well … you get this cluster of symptoms that will last anywhere between one and fifty-five years. And then at the end of it, your bones will hollow out and you'll die tinier." And you press them for details, "What symptoms?" "Well, they're vaguely exactly like all the cancers. But good luck getting that checked out because I have to cure erectile dysfunction again, okay?"'

– Hannah Gadsby

CONTENTS

★BONUS SYMPTOMS★

PREHEAT

Billions of women, generation after generation, enter perimenopause with a resounding '*WHAT?!*' Maybe their hair slinks down the drain, or their tempers flare for the first time, or their arms crawl with phantom spiders. Then they are advised, under billions of breaths, that it's The Change, and they wonder, 'Why didn't anybody tell me?!'

Call me crazy, and you would if this were the nineteenth century, but I'd say the answer is misogyny. Mistrust of women's voices, horror of female aging, shame around women's sexuality, and indifference toward health concerns specific to people with uteruses have conspired to muzzle expression, research, and information about menopause.

A number of books have recently appeared that refuse this received ideology and gather what science there is to help us understand the storm in our bodies and navigate therapeutic options.

This is not one of those books, despite the sciencey subtitle. *Steamy* is part memoir, part nonfiction, part fancy, and part the 'involuntary laughter' an eighteenth-century physician observed in women whose periods had stopped. The symptomology, a list of symptoms, offered me a way to explore the dozens of surprises we encounter in midlife.

One symptom, the hot flash, has escaped silencing, probably because it's a little hard to ignore. You may have witnessed your steaming mother lay down her fork, fling open the front door, and dive into the snow. Perhaps your aunt used to drive with her head out the window like a dog, tongue a windsock. Or maybe the hot flash computes because everybody knows what it feels like to overheat and perspire, so they believe they can relate. They don't all really know, though, how it feels to cremate your own innards like a self-cleaning oven.

If you search these days, you will find many lists of menopause symptoms: 10, 34, 65, even 120 Symptoms of Menopause. While the wildly divergent counts unsettle me a bit, it's encouraging to see the experiences named; unfortunately, many medical practitioners have gone straight from disregarding what patients report to overlooking unrelated health crises. Because if you are a middle-aged woman, everything befalling you – bleeding from the eyes, an arm hanging out of its socket, exploding spleen – is now 'just the menopause.' Nature's way, don't worry about it.

Every person will receive a unique loot bag of symptoms. Very few get all 3,700. Anyone who does deserves a lifetime supply of ice-cream sandwiches and an all-expenses-paid trip to one of those spas with the cold plunge pools. Some folks experience no symptoms at all aside from the end of menstruation. These people deserve to pay for the other guy's ice cream and spa holiday.

I write from the Point Pelee peninsula, which pokes down like a thorn in the side of Lake Erie. I am frequently the southernmost woman in Canada. My home stands next to a marsh, among sassafras trees and python-gauge vines and skinks and possums and fish flies, on the lowest concession road of Leamington, Ontario, the 'tomato capital,' fast becoming the cannabis capital. I wear earplugs to bed in the spring because there's no break between the night-trilling peepers and horny-morning warblers. In other words, I live in a hothouse, which you'd think would have prepared me. Also, I'm a doctor, though not the kind to be of much use here, unless you've got dangling modifiers or an involuted novel. Still, I hope *Steamy* proves some kind of tonic for anyone embarking on this life transition that rattles, zaps, inflames, befuddles, plumps, emboldens, irritates, and somehow wets and dries at the same time.

I wrote this book because one day I said '*WHAT?!*' and *WHAT?!*'s call for investigation. More compelling, though, was the chorus of *WHAT?!*'s surging around me. My friends found themselves in the same position, sucker-punched by a sweaty fistful of symptoms they couldn't believe no one had warned them about. This is for them and for the billions of other hot-and-bothereds out there.

1. LOSS OF FERTILITY

I'm pregnant. My fly won't zip up, stomach acid geysers up through my esophageal sphincter, and the lilac-sweet scent of fresh laundry inspires me to barf in the basket. Happy, happy day!

Then I wake up. I've had this dream since I developed the ability to reproduce. Before I was ever actually pregnant, my unconscious didn't supply gastrointestinal realism, but my reactions were always the same: to the dream pregnancy (thrilled) and to waking up (bummed).

Of course, motherhood is not for everyone, and I know my enthusiasm for it is profoundly boring, but what are you going to do. Be grateful I'm not showing you photos.

When I was a girl I didn't have a dolly. I had eight. I swaddled and coddled them in eight four-quart fruit baskets, lined up cozily under my bedroom window where they could enjoy the natural light. One baby may have been a leopard piggy bank, but all God's creatures and all that. Essentially, I oversaw a maternity ward. You're not supposed to have favourites but as they're all perimenopausal now, and also made of plastic, it's safe to say I loved Brenda the most. She had long mahogany hair and rad chunky bangs, which is weird for a newborn, but she really had me wrapped around her baby finger – no small feat given it was fused to the rest of her hand.

I never had Barbie dolls because of my mother's conviction that dolls should be baby dolls, that their purpose was to prepare you for mothering. She considered Barbie as a kid's plaything a little gross. She had a point: Barbie's prototype was a gentlemen's novelty toy from Germany, an escort doll touted as '*immer diskret*' ('always discreet'). But, to be honest, as much as I loved my babies, I also dug going over to my friends' houses to stage all manner of depraved scenarios with their mini-adults. My pastel nursery didn't supply the frisson of Ken naked handstanding intertwinedly with Growing Hair Cher, the red-track-suited Six Million Dollar Man teetering stiffly on a sack of marbles nearby, watching with his wonky bionic eye. You could share in Steve Austin's wide-angle vision by looking through a hole in the back of his head. Some days this was preferable to the hole Brenda peed through into Kleenex and Scotch-tape diapers when I gave her an empty glue bottle full of apple juice. I guess as a child I was part Michelle Duggar, part German douchebag.

As a very young woman, the disappointment I felt upon waking unpregnant was tempered by the thought that I should probably wait to procreate until I mastered quadratic equations and packed my own lunch. Also, Brenda was still in the room, abandoned at the back of the closet under a mouldering science fair project. She could be diverted only so much by the smudged hypothesis that purple food colouring travels faster through the phloems of celery than the xylems of carnations. A new baby could only add insult to injury.

As an adult I had the dream at least once a month – wait, once a month? Oh, eggs, you really pull all the strings, don't you? The dreams stopped only briefly, during my for-real pregnancy and early parenthood. Then they started up again, proposing little siblings. I was forty-six before I could bear to agree to a procedure that would curb my increasingly generous blood donations (see 3. Cessation of Menses) but turn my womb into a gourd rattle.

Yet the dreams continue. Now they are conundrum dreams. Should I keep it? Could I do it? Dawn Brooke of Guernsey conceived naturally at fifty-eight, and in countries where it's legal, women have used IVF to start families well into their seventies. Imagine having a mom and grandma in one! One hand offering you carrot sticks and hummus, the other tucking a sticky clump of ribbon candy into your pencil case.

The last time I had the dream – triplets mind you, and conceived because I ate an unripe mango, although Jimmy Smits was there – I woke up relieved. I think I'm done. I shall continue to smother my only child with enough love for seven babies and a leopard, and hope all her dreams come true.

I mean, not *all*, obviously. I couldn't afford that much ribbon candy.

2. HOT FLASHES

When I was in my thirties, a student wrote on a teacher-evaluation form that I was 'amazingly hot' and another asked 'could she be any hotter?' Now I have reached my fifties and the answer is Yes! I could be hotter and I am, sometimes every fifteen minutes. Chili peppers would confetti me these days if ratemyprofessors.com hadn't disallowed them.

Because I am so hot. I am so amazingly, stupendously hot I have to keep a hand-held fan in every room. If I can't find a fan, your essay 'Playing with Fire: Pyrogenic Imagery in William Blake's "The Tyger"' will do. If I'm in my bedroom I can choose from the couple dozen *New Yorker*s and *People* magazines spangling the night table, floor, and passenger side of the bed. These make great fans. They are all folded backwards in the middle of long-form journalism articles (on the fall of democracy) and Star Tracks photo-spreads (on the rise of Hemsworths) I can't finish because I'm overtired thanks to the intermittent alarm of night sweats (see 4. Night Sweats).

In the eighteenth century, fanning oneself quickly was code for 'I love you.' Being a contemporary lit person, I did not know this until recently. I apologize, Professor Matheson, for coming on so strong. Also, when I dropped my gloves in our hallway, right at the threshold of your open office door, it was only because my fingers foozled, overfull with black cohosh and Timbits. Next time you place your parasol against your left cheek I will take the hint.

They call it The Change, and as with our planet's weather, 'change' proves a more accurate term than warming. Yes, we endure more hot days, but it's the volatility that's dangerous. I am a spitting sparking deep fryer full of breaded brie. Then I am a frosty mug of beer. Then I am that sparking brie again. Over and over. It sounds delicious but it can make one a little hot under the collar. It can make one a cold bitch. It has been suggested that postmenopausal women are the most psychologically tranquil humans, therefore most likely to thrive during lengthy flight in space and exile on Mars. Notice they say *post*menopausal women, not menopausal women. We share temperaments with NHL enforcers. And our mullets get just as sweaty.

One of the Spanish words for hot flash is *bochorno*, which can also mean 'embarrassment.' And if you are pregnant you are *embarazada*. (And if you have a cold you are *constipada* – no wonder I always have so much trouble making myself understood at the *farmacia*.) What's with all the embarrassment? There's no need to draw my fan across my face which, by the way, is another sign for 'I love you.' It has been observed, notably by Enlightenment physicians, that older women spontaneously combust on occasion, but I don't see why that should red-flag my petition to rocket to Mars.

I will thaw your car lock during an ice storm, just by giving it the eye. You can fry an egg on my leg. I will warm up your pizza pockets in my pockets. If there's room. I'm incubating a clutch of endangered piping plover eggs in there. Turn down the thermostat! I forestall climate change by conserving fossil fuels. I just sit there and radiate. I heat up the faculty lounge so fast everybody starts fanning and I'm spoiled for choice.

3. CESSATION OF MENSES

I'm not sure why I never went to the doctor.

Maybe because I was so relieved each time my tsunami ended that I didn't want to think about it again until three weeks later when I ruined the *other* side of the couch cushion.

Maybe because my parents did not go to doctors. I've never heard my tiny mother complain about anything. Breast cancer, life-threatening pneumonia, four children, including nine-pound twins. Each. She's not going to waste time whining. Her bunions have migrated so far her skinny naked feet look like the eyes of the grinning/squinting emoji, and she just straps on her extra-wide sneakers and marches past the dawdlers scaling Mount Whitney.

Maybe it was embarrassment. I was already several years into managing the deluge when censors first allowed the word 'period' to be spoken in a TV commercial, by Courteney Cox in a skim milk–hued leotard.

Maybe because I took it as a given that other people shared my experience. When it comes to things done in private, there's not much opportunity to gauge the norm. I know I was, for example, opening umbrellas pretty much as often as other people and deploying them with similar technique, so why wouldn't the same be true of tampons? My assuming everybody suffers a few days wearing two Super Plus cotton corks and a Mega Size Ruffin' It Lil' Squirts puppy-training mat with wings and staying near a bathroom so they can change them out every forty-five minutes made me kind of like that guy I heard interviewed on the radio who assumed everybody else also had a poop knife, until the day he called out from his buddy's bathroom to ask where he kept his. Didn't all gals have a bad-towel shelf? Dark-jeans week? Contrary to popular belief, women don't constantly discuss their periods with one another, so I didn't really know. When a partner just tucked a couple squares of toilet paper in her pants one afternoon a month, I figured that was just some butch hormone phenomenon. Opposites attract. I understand some women catch their period in a wee silicone bowl tucked up the cooch. Barista! I'll have a venti passionberry frappe, with beet milk, and please pour it into this doll's teacup!

My life's menstrual misadventures are legion. On a day trip with the in-laws when I was twenty-three I went to the bathroom at every stop, no matter how outsized and grubby the gas station keychain, just to check. I knew the vermillion tide would be rolling in soon and toted around a backpack stuffed with absorbent paraphernalia. By the end of the day, nothing had materialized, so on the ride home I let myself doze off on the powder-blue upholstery of my father-in-law's about-to-be-sold Corolla. Yep.

At swim practice, cherry Kool-Aid rivulets braided down my inner thighs. And that was after doubling up on the white dynamite. My friend Jen had recently advised me that nothing comes out when you're swimming in the pool, because of water pressure or whatever. Remember the cloud haloing that dumped chum bucket in *Jaws*?

Then there was me perched on the toilet at twelve, holding my breath while my mother shaved down an o.b. tampon, put Vaseline on it and, after my own flustered attempts, *inserted it for me* while the swim team carpool honked in the driveway. Many of the indignities involve swim team. A confident lady in a white bikini and/or on a white horse with beach-tousled hair I was not.

When I picture myself between twelve and fifty-two, I see a woman with a cartoon vampire permanently latched to her neck. Whether I was unsuccessfully dodging balls in the junior-high gym, sweating through a polyester blazer during my first university lecture, or getting trounced in a game of Candyland with my three-year-old, I always carried this popped-collar loser tossed over one shoulder. My John Hancock is embarrassingly minimalist, a sidewalk-dried worm, and that's not thanks to youthful affectation but rather the grave anemia draining my signature-developing years.

So why do I miss my monthly pain in the ass?

It has something to do with rhythm. I've lived in a couple of different equatorial countries and that was an adventure and everything, but I missed the dramatic morphing of seasons. The sky sparkled and the breeze loosed the fragrance of sexy ruffled flowers every day of the year and that was sort of depressing. Not the short-term yet deeply lacerating kind of depressing specific to a Canadian January when the Seasonal Affective Disorder drives you out into the freeze to lick at the weak white sun for as many minutes as you can stand while your extremities drop off. That's almost pleasurable: the keener the nadir, the more ecstatic the green gush of geosmin-scented spring to follow. No, living without seasons dealt merely a mild chronic horror at the prospect of time as a line rather than a looping thread. No *hello hello again* to dragonfly fleets, then scrolling red leaves, then squeaky crystals under the boots, then muddy bunnies chewing tulip heads.

And maybe it's because I had it so bad. Many things have fallen away with age, but the one I miss most is the one that caused me the greatest aggravation. It's not the tranquil and velvetsoft Persian cat but the cantankerous, incontinent, burr-encrusted tom who leaves a gaping void when he dies.

Aristotle noted that when a menstruating woman looks in a mirror, it clouds over. Period blood can also kill locusts and, during an eclipse, men. I miss that!

I could follow the advice of Hippocrates and stimulate my cycle by making a pessary of myrrh, alum, beef bile, and dung.

Did you have to look up 'pessary'? Think tampon. Beef-bile tampon.

On the other hand, now I don't have to pack a bad towel to protect white hotel sheets, I can spend my money in the marshmallow aisle rather than the so-called feminine hygiene aisle, and I revel in the new-found muscle power born of iron retention. I can now stretch at the barre in a skim-milk leotard (I mean I *could*). I am impregnable.

Did you have to look up 'geosmin'? It was worth it, I hope, to identify the compound that delivers the heady perfume of awakening soil in March. Apparently, humans can detect it more successfully than sharks can smell blood in the water.

4. NIGHT SWEATS

It's not so bad, 3 a.m., a warm dew, an unexpected airplane hot towel. I wipe the pretzel dust off my fingers. My cat snuggles up because he likes the heat, purrs a quickly dripping tap. Now it's a eucalyptus steam, soothing. Soothing at first, but starting to cloy. How do the other women breathe in here, in this half-lucid dream where I am the only one not starkers and that's so humiliating. I kick down the duvet. Now I bead, I puddle, and every few minutes I tug at my T-shirt, as if I can dry it by flapping it away from and back to my sternum a few times like a boyband boy telling my ceiling fan how much I love it, out of my chest my huge runny heart thump-thump-thump-kathwacks (see 26. Palpitations), and now it's a full-on wet T-shirt contest and I didn't win but I got a special prize for filling my own pail, the judge is my ceiling fan who, hoping for nips, enthusiastically cools the sweat, colds it, frigids it, and now I am Kate Winslet slogging and keening through the lower decks, shouting *Jack Jack Jack*, waist-deep in icy Atlantic waters, my sweat goes sub-zero, I'm Kate on the floating door, Edwardian skirts ice-stiffened, death swimming my way, I peel off my T-shirt and fling it across the dark sea, pull the beach back up over both of us, me and Leo, that's my cat.

5. MOOD SWINGS™

They look like ordinary swings, rubberized U's that cinch your hips like a pebble in a fiercely drawn slingshot.

Shuffle your feet in the sand to get started and then lean back and stick your legs out straight. The sunny park whooshes slightly.

Then lean forward and bend your knees as you slip backwards into a bit of a letdown.

Then find your gumption and yank on the chains and kick your legs out again and this isn't half bad. Then lean forward and air-squat and slide back, noting the dark, pocked dirt beneath you, a cigarette butt.

Then chain-yank and snap your legs out into the joyful throes of sky and there's a croissant-shaped cloud (a *chocolate* croissant!). Then forward bend, slide back, sand squirms in your shoes and the screeching of the rusty metal shackles above you is maybe the saddest sound in the world. Then stretch back and power forward and you yourself have created the balmy wind flicking jubilantly through your hair, then scrunch over and fall back because what is your purpose on this earth anyway, then kick out, and whee up into seventh heaven. Maybe you can gather so much momentum you will nail a full circle around the top beam!

Slip backwards, and the full-moon end of the butt filter is stained something between yellow and brown, baby-poo colour, probably why they call it a butt. Launch forward, you will *definitely* make it all the way around. Retreat, realize you have made a terrible mistake, twisting out on a wobbly limb, inches away from bashing your head on the side post. But you are a playground wizard, flying forward again, ratcheting up that amplitude with every exultant pendulum arc. Even though the duration of each oscillation – in physics that's called a period! – increases, it feels like slap-happy time is about to do a loop-de-loop with you.

Swing back and down and backwards-up and dread the weightless second of suspension at the turnaround point before gravity sucks your stupid body forward-down again, leaving your uterus to continue wandering up by itself just as the ancient Greek physician Aretaeus said it would, and this is it, this is the time you'll round the top bar like the International Space Station circling the earth, like a bucket of water whipped around so fast not a drop falls out. You're there, you're seriously almost there! And then something goes awry and you are not the ISS or a bucket and you hear the groans and clangs of cascading chains and you're flying solo now, dripping wax, sinking into a sea of sand.

Above you the squeaks abate. On the underside of your swing there is a small block of white text, peeling but legible:

MOOD SWING™ COLOUR KEY

RED passionate, ready for romance
ORANGE adventure, possible reckless, YOLO!
YELLOW mellow or sleepy / boring
GREEN optimism and friendly
BLUE bliss
INDIGO bad day in the office?
VIOLET howling abyss of wretchedness

Struggle to your knees and grab the seat for a look. You left a rainbow.

6. CHILLS

I trumble my shopping cart out of the Superstore, sauntering into the parking lot without a reliable mental screenshot of where I left the car. A guy walks toward me, about fifty feet away, casually leering in that male-gazey way. It's been a while.

In undergraduate Spanish class, to which I wore flowing flour-sack tent dresses, gaze-deflecting and pleasingly soft against the legs, I sat *incrédula* at my brilliant and merry grey-haired professor who assured us that while we may feel irritated now by relentless catcalling in the streets of Barcelona, when we got to a certain age we would relish it.

Now I am that certain age. Am I relishing this? Be honest. Can someone mostly in the lesbian zone of the sexuality spectrum, and well versed in the cultural tyranny of patriarchal surveillance (I'm talking to you, wiener-dog-walking creep who clapped in my face today because I avoided eye contact while jogging past), get some weird ginseng slurp to the ego from being considered cute by some dick in a parking lot? Now that decades of life experience have rendered me a little less porous, can I occasionally enjoy a desiring gaze?

Kinda.

But of course it's not a purely desiring gaze. It's an appraising gaze, as becomes obvious when he gets a bit closer and can see me a bit more clearly, and he drops that gaze. A beat of horror slackens his facial muscles, like *Oh shit, it's an old lady!*

Can someone who has a PhD and publishes books of feminist poetry and has plenty of loving in her life and could pull this guy's asshole out through his ear in a game of Scrabble be made to feel for an instant like a silky ermine in winter woods that turns out upon closer inspection to be a ragged length of toilet paper on the forest floor?

Kinda.

Anyway, I found my car. And I've related this encounter to a few friends, trying especially to capture that flash of revulsion on the man's face, and it's a funny story, kinda.

7. FINE LINES AND WRINKLES

One morning in the mid-oughts, my computer greeted me with an array of cremation urns I could purchase for a loved one, some ornately carved, some sleek and contemporary like a hotel ice bucket. The selection included ash containers for every budget, from $59.95 to latest iPhone. To encounter this information seemed bizarre enough, and then I realized I had brought the advertising on myself. This was my introduction to internet data collection; the day before, I had been looking for images of classical artifacts to accompany my lecture on Keats's 'Ode on a Grecian Urn.'

Now I'm more likely to be targeted with urns for my own remains. When I hit my fiftieth birthday, the Ontario government sent me a mammogram reminder and a plastic toothpick I was to poke at my feces with and send back to them. So it's not surprising the digital universe also knows how old I am, and it seems really concerned I'm going to forget.

I could be scrolling through social media, checking out my niece's adorable cowboy costume or collegially popping a heart onto somebody's frolicking Pomeranian video while Leo gives me the side-eye, and the next thing I know the feed is shouting *You are made entirely of crepe paper! Do something!* My online investigations and diversions are regularly screen-bombed by ads warning me my bones will snap, my hair will go mangy, my back will U-turn over, and my inadequate life insurance will leave my child to make meals out of dandelion greens and cloudy basement-pickles.

But I have to admit to succumbing to the most powerful arm of the anti-aging propaganda machine: the skin-care routine. You don't wash your face; you practise a regimen. It involves multiple steps and old-timey apothecary bottles and finger-circling motions, and you're not supposed to get any of it in your eyes, especially the eye cream. You've got to run a rose quartz paint roller up and down your cheeks with the zeal of a fanless band wheatpasting gig flyers. You must use the L-ascorbic acid serum. That's Tang for your face! Don't skip the hyaluronabananic acid. SPF 2000. Squooges of aloe. Organic eyes of newts. Not that I'm anti-collagen but what is *Pro* Collagen? You might become so irresistible after layering on all these unguents that somebody will want to lick your shiny face and lustfully exclaim 'Phlbleh!'

When as a young woman I'd find myself in the bathroom of a friend's middle-aged mom, I'd look at the prismatic display of expensive potions and think *What a scam!*, and then my pal and I would microwave Velveeta nachos and drink a bottle of Malibu coconut rum and smoke mouldy hash and go out dancing till 4 a.m., puke a little, collapse for a couple hours and wake up smooth and dewy as organic newts. But a while ago I simultaneously hit menopause and endured the harrowing dissolution of a twenty-year partnership. In a year I aged like a two-term American president. At the end of it I looked in the mirror at the fine lines and wrinkles and wondered if I should Benjamin Button myself, try to figure out what a retinoid is.

Then I considered my own mother. In a pandemic January, seniors queued up outside the Costco at 8 a.m.,

Canadianly six feet apart, snugly toqued and stamping their boots on the rock-salted blacktop. An employee surveyed the crowd and shouted at my mum, 'Hey, this is for seniors only, you'll have to wait for regular hours!' My gentle-natured tiny mother ripped off her hat, revealing fluffy white hair, and proclaimed, 'Dear, I am eighty years old!' to a long line of mittened applause. The same week, a deferential, Smurf-haired cashier at Shoppers Drug Mart asked me if I would like to take advantage of the senior's discount. Yes Dear, I would, actually, like to take advantage of it — a little payback for being mistaken for a decade older than I am.

So while other people might balk at the furrowed cheeks of the previous generation and amass an arsenal of age-defying creams and serums and makeup to forestall the same, I look to my mother, whose cosmetics collection consists of one tube of lips-coloured lipstick (purchased at Canadian Tire) (for weddings) and hope I can inherit something more than my dawning habit of calling everyone *Dear*.

8. BRAIN FROG

Brain frog is a very common symptom of perimenopause and menopause, and many women say that their brains feel as if stuffed with kitten world. You might have noticed that you are increasingly forgetful, can't remember gnomes, lose your keister, write endless tada! lists, become confusedly easy, and find it hard to remain in formation. This can make it especially hard to function a twerk, and you might juggle to concentrate when reeking or washing TV.

These symptoms can be so severe that you may even start to worry that you have de munchies. This is particularly scary if you have a foamy hysteria, and some women become so concerned that they are refried for tasting at a mummery clinic. Fortunately, the right type and dose of homo replacement threnody (HRT) (with Toblerone for those who need it) can improve brain frog and help you thunk more clunkly.

9. INSOMNIA

Did I eat too much dark chocolate? Did I set the alarm to a.m.? Did I concede enough? Was I assertive enough? Did the soup have MSG in it? Is two hours of sleep restorative? Are my telomeres shrinking? Too assertive? Does my living space seem cheery to me but kind of grimy to other people? Should I open the door for a cross-breeze? Are the seams of my brokenness fused with gold? Or busy with pocked grit and quackgrass? When did I last change the furnace filter? What time is it? Should I get up and do crunches? Do dark circles make me look haggard? Or sexy? With the first faint colourlift of dawn could I walk without fear? Even though I have to buy the lightweight kitty litter, could my lifetime of pent-up resentment knock out an attacker? Did I leave my charger in Guelph? If I lie still will my Restless Leg Syndrome subside? Theoretically speaking, could I be a great-great-grandmother? Was that a thud or a thump? 90210: Where are they now? A spray of pebbles or a groan?

What time is it? What is the weather in Northumberland, PA? Should I have asked him to repeat himself instead of laughing as if I had heard? Would I rather drown in a pool of custard or be hunted down by a bear? Did I chuckle instead of answering a question? Would they kill the bear or could it lumber away to safety? Would they drain the custard? Could I be a father? What's that in Celsius? What is the point of me? Can I hold it until morning? Did he ask the way to the highway and I went *heh heh* as if to say 'Wouldn't you like to know'? Could a fur-matted furnace filter catch fire? What's so inspirational about *Dead Poets Society*? INT. CAVE – NIGHT. GLORIA: Yeah. If you guys don't have a meeting, how do we know if we wanna join? NEIL: *Join?!* What time is it? Aren't Emily Dickinson and Gertrude Stein also dead? What time is it? Am I impossible? You up?

10. LACK OF MOTIVATION

My daughter – let's call her Elise (we said, in 2004) – has a lot of plans and, thanks to teenage circadian rhythms, she likes to discuss them long past the hour when my own mind has gone fuzzy and still, a curled-up old cat you check to confirm it's still breathing. In the interests of bonding, I'll sit up in my bed – yes, sometimes with my eyes closed – as she leans against my knees and deliberates over which make of grand piano will grace the top landing of her expansive spiral staircase with the hand-carved balusters and where the upright pianos will go and whether or not an electronic piano would suffice for the home office. There are many features to discuss, from pool grottoes to jewel-tone paint colours to number of biological and adopted children, the only constant being the shit-ton of pianos and Tony awards. I am down with it all, especially the Arts and Crafts–style granny cottage out by the grotto.

I hum along with her energy. Children restore the super-saturation to Santa, lure you back to the floor to build Lego towns, and give you an excuse to bake and eat over-frosted cupcakes. They also orient perspective forward again, toward what could happen rather than what's gone down.

During one of our gab sessions she proposed we name our hopes and dreams for the next five, the next ten, the next twenty years. Her agenda is fully fleshed out, from the smash-hit musicals she will compose and perform in, to the husband with wavy dark hair who is prettier than her but not smarter, equally talented but in a slightly different area. Then she asked me about my hopes and dreams.

This was a daytime heart-to-heart, in the car on a not-busy country highway, leaving no excuse for not participating. But I found myself stymied. And also, in the honeyed light of a June afternoon, a bit dark-night-of-the-soul. All my life I'd galloped along on hope dream hope dream plan strategize hope dream. I always knew what new thing I wanted my five-years-older self to be doing. Now I couldn't think. My daughter fiddled with her Spotify queue and a Tupperware container while I meditated upon it … I got nothing. Was that my gusto in the rear-view mirror, tumbling off into the ditch?

Elise handed me a grape. Sunlight shot through the translucent blob, and I popped that glowing purple planet into my mouth. And I thought *Hey, I do not burble over with hopes and dreams anymore because so many that I used to have came true.* At thirty I was still keeping an eye to the sidewalk on the off chance I'd find change for the laundromat. Now I live in a farmhouse among the trees I planted twenty years ago so I could exist among trees, with books on the shelf, some with my name on the spine, an old cat I have to check for breathing, and a piano. And the one thing I wanted more than anything, this dreamer who asked me the question in the first place.

P.S. Okay, I wrote that a couple of years ago. My daughter is still and forever my favourite planet, but since then I decided to make this book about menopause, started piano lessons, and saw the mostly cool Barbie movie where I was supposed to tear up (see 29. Dry Eyes) at purportedly the film's most moving and profound idea that 'mothers stand still so our daughters can look back to see how far they have come.' Um, what? (See 37. Bloating.) (See 41. Individuation.) (See 45. Fewer Shits.) Bitch, I'm not standing still.

11. ANXIETY

(See 39. Anxiety.)

12. VISION PROBLEMS

I no longer have just one pair of glasses. I have glasses

for driving
for reading
for riving
for dreading
for just normal life
for just normal life through the top and reading
this medication may cause blurred vision through the bottom
for making out street signs through the top and folding
maps through the bottom. folding maps?! born before disco
and contact lenses
much?
for making out
for sheet music though the piano keys are blurry
for keys though the music is blurry
for looking down through and then up over
for holding an inch out, then lifting a smidge, then throwing aside in favour of naked
crossed eyes
for watching the opening credits of American Horror Story
rose-coloured
cannabis-scented
Sour Patch Kids-flavoured
for seeing what the future holds: surprise, it's more glasses!
for looking chic though I can't see anything
for looking uggo though I can see everything
for spotting a butterfly earring-back at the bottom of a silver pool
for counting the rings of Saturn and naming each midge in a swarm
for naming the Midge
and the second Moose
for looking for your glasses
for looking through the looking glass
for making a 1000-piece Sloths of the Rainforest puzzle half-assedly
for looking at the glass half-assed
for looking for ass in all the wrong places
for looking at it all wrong

13. REDUCED IMMUNE FUNCTION

In early April 2021 the Ontario government declares that those over fifty living in hotspots can register for their COVID vaccine. A few days later I navigate a long empty road through pastoral Essex County, following the temporary signage toward the hockey arena where I will get my shot. Finally, between nowhere and nowhere, a solar-powered dot-matrix LED message board declares:

VACCINATION
CLINIC ENTRANCE

Typo aside, a welcome change from the dystopian Lite-Brites we've been encountering for a year:

BORDER IS CLOSED

STAY AT HOME

TURN BACK!

EAT ANOTHER DOUGH TUBE

SUPPRESS YOUR THROAT TICKLE

DON'T SHOUT 'ARE YOU TRYING TO
KILL EVERYONE?!' AT THE LADY
LINGERING WITH HER NOSE OUT
OVER THE PARSLEY YOU NEED

DO OR DON'T LET YOUR TEENAGER SEE YOU LOSE IT?

YOU HAVEN'T HUGGED YOUR SISTER IN 18 HOPE 19 MONTHS

I advance through the cheerful labyrinth of safety cones and fluorescent-vested volunteers, who invite me after every turned corner to take a pump of diamond-clear Hope Glop. Everybody rubs their gloppy hands together as we file along. We are a congregation of gleeful conspirators, pestilence-spreading flies. I have been so well trained to keep my two-metre distance from others that when I arrive at the nurse with the needles I instinctively drag the proffered chair away from her. She snatches it back, a little irritated (I'm not the first) (see 24. Irritability), motions for me to sit, and proceeds to ask me a dozen questions, close as pillow talk, close enough for me to read her name tag. In some terrible irony, am I going to catch the virus from Silke, the very person trying to protect me from it? Couldn't she somehow jab me at arm's length? Could she not have infused the mRNA into a gummy dart and tossed it at my open mouth from across the clinio?

A fluorescent teenager marshals me toward floor arrows, which marshal me to a sanitized monobloc where I must wait fifteen minutes for hives and wheezing. The arena holds an expansive grid of mid-lifers, creating a Quilt of Wisdom, or Faded Bloom Acre. It's mostly orderly, aside from the forest-camo dude in front of me who at the five-minute mark starts snorting incredulously and lifting his meaty upturned palms in a plea for everyone to acknowledge the outrageous inconvenience of it all. Harbinger of the national temper tantrum to come.

These are my peers on display, organized into two-metre-square installations. Many sit in cozy twos. When signing up online, you had to choose 'Single' or 'Couple.' (Lori and I split up years ago, but you don't realize when you first divorce that the little jabs to the heart never stop – the end never-ending). While this outing may not prove the most romantic of dates, neither does it offer a very appealing singles mixer. I see no lesbians, at least not the visibly butch kind I go for. No dykey swaggers, no hints of womanly curve under masculine duds, no rings of keys. Most of the people resemble Mr. Impatient, and I'm not about to spend my life scrambling to find my wallet and gloves while my husband leans on the horn in the driveway.

There's nothing like sitting in an exhibit of your age cohort to make you wish you hadn't eaten those tubes of cookie dough and prompt you to consider training for a half-marathon. Not a whole marathon, because come on. But at least something that will keep you limber long enough that you're still around when it's time to start calling you *spry*. I want to turn around and climb back up that hill I'm over.

Thank you, Silke, for giving me the shot in the arm I needed.

14. MEMORY LOSS

Who is that actor, the Cleveland boyfriend of Liz Lemon who coached English football and whom I pitied whenever I heard 'Watermelon Sugar'? What's that dish steamed in corn husks? Who did that song 'We Like to Party'? What was the name of that delish licorice gum? What was the name of that candy shop on Highway 11 where we got it? What was that book by that guy from the place?

Do you feel it takes longer to retrieve the terms you're looking for these days? For me I'm not sure it's that much worse than it ever was. My neural connections have always wobbled and juddered with perching and launching birds, but when you reach midlife you attribute lapses to aging.

Proper names are the worst, because of their arbitrariness. All language is arbitrary, but at least once we've settled on the word *fruit*, we can agree on the category (tomatoes, I know I know). But what a Paul is, that's just not a secure category. You may say every Paul you know is a wanker, and therefore you know the 'meaning' of Paul, but perhaps I know a nice one. Wait, bad example.

Let me help. Rather than submitting to promising new experiments like innervating your anterior temporal lobes by means of transcranial direct current stimulation to the scalp, you can exercise your memory with this Word Search:

```
J A S O N S I E V E K I S T
O N I C B I F F B X I P N H
L T R U D O L L Y B L A K E
E A Q V E V P A U L L S B C
N M U G R E E T C A D U A A
E A R L G R E Y C C E Z N N
S L O A O H W M A K E I U D
I E S X N A E D M B R E S Y
E S S I E V E N G A B O Y S
V O Z R R E M E I R T Y S I
E A D U I P I P I F G O Y E
C N W A L M A R M ? N G M V
A S I L A Y S I E V I N G E
```

15. VAGINAL DRYNESS

Do you really think I would tell you if I have vaginal dryness? I have students. We devour the radical honesty of memoir, don't we, but eughy. If I have vaginal dryness or vaginal wetness – either way I lose. Either way I'm the elementary school teacher whose students are shocked to see buying peanut butter at Zehrs. Crunchy *or* smooth. But so much worse than that.

How can the most reviled word in the English language be 'moist' and the most shameful symptom of menopause 'vaginal dryness'? It's the cherry on top of that heap of can't-win paradoxes of womaning under patriarchy. Dried or soaked in maraschino syrup.

What even is vaginal dryness? How can a vagina be dry? When my doctor was listing off menopause symptoms I stopped him there. 'You mean, like, relatively, right?' 'Yes, relatively,' he replied dryly. Similarly, dry mouth (see 36. Dry Mouth) is not literally dry. A dry martini is not literally dry. You will never tip an empty glass of nothing but a desiccated olive into your desert woodrat nest of a mouth.

Vaginal dryness is one of the bouquet of symptoms that comes with 'vaginal atrophy', another evocative term which, while replaced in 2014 by GSM (Genitourinary Syndrome of Menopause), is still a great favourite with physicians. (They also can't quit 'incompetent cervix'.)

I will tell you, because I'm not embarrassed to mortify my poor teenaged self, that when I came of age I didn't know anything about moistness. In the late seventies, Sex Ed had nothing to say about the physiological manifestations of female desire. That's why, after Colin gave me a back massage on his rec room floor, I was sure I had soaked the harvest gold shag with blood (see 3. Cessation of Menses) or, bewilderingly, pee (see 20. Urinary Incontinence).

16. DEPRESSION

I try to cultivate the attitude that when the yard is full of shit there must be a pony, but after decades of life, a hormonal low yields a carousel of hollowing memories – some even featuring actual ponies. Don't worry, no ponies die.

Cool September morning at the county fair; the attendant perched preschoolers on the pony, doggedly circling a post at the end of its tether. We inched forward with the other parents, and tots in turn gaspgiggled and thrilled at their first ride. I was relieved to see another animal chewing hay under a dusty awning. They would spell each other off. The attendant charmed the families, polite to the parents and indulgent with the kids. 'Say "horsey" – Mom's taking your picture,' 'Look at your awesome cowboy hat!' 'Hold on tight, little lady!'

We were also just a family at the fair. Just parents hoping our dimpled little two-year-old would gigglegasp at riding a pony on a cool September morning. Our turn came and the attendant placed our daughter on the brittle leather saddle, a jagged glint flaring up in his eyes, now trained on us rather than her. He was one of those Flannery O'Connor characters at the moment the evil slides out.

'You two sisters?' He steadied her but Elise looked a little unsure.

As was I about what to answer. 'Something like that?'

He tugged at the animal, stumbling over its clops, so he could round back to us more quickly. 'Oh, well I'm groovy with it. I'm not the kind to judge anybody.' He straightened our solemn toddler on her wobbling perch without looking at her. The pony plodded. 'I don't know why people have a problem with it.' A mosquito bite swelling the thin baby-skin above Elise's barely-there eyebrow. 'If you ever need someone to join in, I'm okay with it. I don't have a problem with it at all. I'm really more than fine with it actually.'

I retreated a few steps, projected several *Great job*s at Elise, and waited for the coiling to stop. The dads and moms behind me also waited, placid, confident appropriate decorum would return for those who deserved it.

It's many years later now, and fall, and the yard is filling up.

The tree outside my window shits apples.

By the end of the day the bite had closed our baby's eye.

17. BURNING MOUTH SYNDROME

Burning Mouth Syndrome?

This is not on the standard shortlist of symptoms. But when my mouth was burning and I googled it, I read that a flaming gob can be a consequence of folate deficiency or high tastebud density or diabetes or, you know, menopause.

This is the way menopause sneaks more symptoms in, by piggybacking on innumerable other conditions. Sore wrists? Could be carpal tunnel. Or menopause. Tinnitus? Too much drumming, or menopause. Facial tic, leg bent the wrong way, overabundance of snot? Menopause, menopause, menopause.

Couldn't they come up with a better name than Burning Mouth Syndrome? I'm not sure why some conditions get all the Latin. My pigmentation disorder has two awesome, legit-sounding names: *leukoderma* and *vitiligo* – take your pick! (I prefer *vitiligo* because it sounds like it could find you a flight to Cabo San Lucas for under $200 or rouse a droopy midlife libido).

But then I'm like 'Doc, my legs feel all restless' and they're like 'There's a name for that – it's called Restless Leg Syndrome. *And it's a symptom of menopause.*'

18. DIZZY SPELLS

'You came to the ER during a pandemic.' I think the doctor is irritated? (See 24. Irritability.) I hit my head way too hard but because I didn't lose consciousness they say it is not technically a concussion. I keep saying, 'Something's screwy,' but that doesn't give them much to go on. How do I explain it? It's not pain (yet) but I feel like an old comic-book page misaligned in the printing, where the tortoise is green in the middle but yellow rises out of its back and cyan seeps below. My tortoise baseball cap is overlapping circles of yellow and magenta like the Mastercard logo. They ask me to walk a line on the floor but I move out of register with the body that is adequately doing it, with the little rubber doll feet a mile down there, apparently mine. I leave with an information sheet about watching for vomiting and combative behaviour. Parking cost seventeen dollars. Barf. Why I oughta!

I had gotten up at barely dawn just for a pee (see 20. Urinary Incontinence), attempting to stay partly asleep while doing so in order that I might stave off morning. This was my habit – keep the lights off, one eye closed – and though of late I tottered a bit during these half-conscious excursions, I never imagined falling down. I was a Weeble, or a used-car-lot tube man. But that morning I did trip and plummet and smash my cerebellum on the hardwood arm of the hardwood bench I had recently hauled up the stairs because I thought it would look cool in my bathroom. Also useful, like if somebody needed to consult me while on the toilet.

After a couple days of birthing-Athena-out-of-my-head pain and visits to doctors who assure me I'll be fine by the weekend, the not-technically-a-concussion fully blooms. Any activity that involves moving through space becomes gruelling. For a while I do everyday things because I believe I'll feel better any second now. But the grocery store contorts into a funhouse mirror maze, and driving gives me an acute burnout sensation. I travel ten minutes and have to turn back because my brain starts to rumble and hiss, threatening to spew shrapnel. By the time I hit the welcoming crunch of my own driveway, smoke tendrils out the car windows.

I take matters into my own hands and find a YouTube video called Yoga for Concussion. I have never done yoga. I thought it was only for dog people who like kombucha and can at least touch their knees. Concussion yoga demands sitting comfortably and turning your head slowly from side to side, keeping your eyes fixed on the raised finger of your choice. Also moving that finger from side to side and following it with your eyeballs. I crush concussion yoga.

Maybe it is a placebo, but the yoga makes me feel a bit better. I want to sense I am doing *something* to combat this Terrible, Horrible, No Good, Very Bad feeling. Exercising even a smidgen of agency can upend a mountain. During childbirth, the giant grey ball in the birthing room meant for inducing labour proved for me the ticket to surviving it. I sat on that squishy-firm moon, facing the mattress with arms resting before me, and when a contraction came I rolled forward, a total of about two millimetres.

It didn't matter how far I moved, the point was that I met the pain, acting rather than enduring, subject rather than object. Many years before that, it turned out that my 'freshman fifteen' (see 34. Weight Gain) was actually an ovarian tumour. Here's where I first learned this agency trick and here's also where friends come in. How could I wait two weeks for surgery, aware there was an ever-expanding alien in my gut, ready to bust through my flesh and kill John Hurt, or me? Knowing it was absurd but knowing I needed it anyway, I called the woowooest person I knew and asked if she had any tinctures or potions that would fight cancer. She chose that day to lay some logic on me: 'You know, Susan, that's not going to fix it.' Hours later, without prompting, my least woowoo friend, Nicole, who knew surgery was the only answer and knew that I and everybody else knew that, brought me a present, a box of something dubiously and wonderfully called Anti-Cancer Tea. And every day after that until my surgery, she brought me another present: Snakes and Ladders, a pineapple, a kazoo. Some people are just healers.

I got off topic there (see 40. Difficulty Concentrating). Back to tortoises. Another friend, Michelle, calls me from Alberta to talk to me in my concussion bed. She is also a professor and understands that while I'm not flaking on teaching, because I'm on sabbatical, I feel anxious about the research I'm supposed to be doing but can't because words keep sliding off the page. But of course the real agenda of sabbaticals, for which professors can apply every seven years, is to handle life. Your sabbatical application might as well read: *For the first few months I plan to suffer a death in the family. While grief continues to erode my energies and hope, I will embark on a calamitous health episode and a divorce (both of which were partly brought on by the last six years of academic life). If time allows, I will deliver my years of research up a pump hose after my basement floods.* In other words, everybody on Earth needs a sabbatical. Michelle also knows about brain-fry, having experienced a stroke. She gives me the image that conveys perfectly how I feel when attempting to navigate the world: a shell-less tortoise.

It's Elise's friend's mom Lisa (see 41. Individuation) who advises me to go to a physiotherapist. Physiotherapists get that you can sustain a concussion without blacking out. They have all the squishy balls and eye-finger exercises you could ever need, and can explain what's going on in your brain. I relearn the basics last acquired in 1969: moving and taking in my surroundings at the same time, because the signals and connections enabling that multitask fritzed out when I hit the bench.

After three months I graduate from the gateway drug of concussion yoga to just plain yoga. I learn that it welcomes cat people. And cow people. I can now walk a tightrope to the bathroom with my eyes closed, hungover, cinching a pineapple between my knees. But I don't. I use the headlamp my friend Andrea sends me.

So, to review, menopause made me a little dizzy, which led to a fall and concussion, which made me critically dizzy, which led me to yoga, which made me dizz-proof. The morals of this chapter serve us well in menopause: Don't roll your eyes when someone extols yoga, unless they wrap an ankle around their own neck while doing it. While expelling Athena out of your head might hurt, you've birthed wisdom and ass-kicking. Friends help keep your shell on.

19. FORMICATION

You read it right. Formication. Could it mean boinking on vintage countertops and kitchen tables? I wish!

But it refers to the sensation of bugs crawling over your arms and legs. Ants, if you're strict about the entomological etymology (and who isn't?). I've experienced this sensation, but that was only because *actual* ants were crawling over my arms and legs.

I've lived long enough now to have witnessed the pencil-sized saplings I planted in my backyard mushroom into a forest. I wanted to create a haven, a wildlife resort, which I envisioned would host warblers and cottontails and cartoon chipmunks. The odd doe-eyed doe would stroll through.

Among those trees I arranged calculatedly to grow in natural random formation, digging out and repositioning any pencil that contributed to a straight row, the deer do amble, lovely and lousy with ticks. Also feeling welcome: rats, skunks, and raccoons, who find they just don't feel comfortable doing number two anywhere but my driveway. At night they dash giddily through the other neighbourhood properties, trying to hold it, debating as they scamper which is harder on the bowels, crayfish or Maltesers wrappers, one of them 'really prairie-doggin' here,' until phew, my driveway, marked now as what raccoon scientists term a 'latrine.' Did you know that raccoon poop often contains the roundworm Baylisascaris procyonis which if accidentally (or on purpose) ingested or inhaled will eat away at your brain?

I'm not going to hurt these guys, so I try calling various animal removal companies. Every one of them features a raccoon photo on the home page of their website. Apparently only because they are so damn cute. (And they really are! Once I aimed a flashlight beam out my tent flap at a raccoon tucking into my marshmallows; instead of running away it just covered its eyes with one hand and with the other continued to dig into the Jet-Puffed Jumbo bag and stuff its muzzle, winsomely foamy with sugar or rabies). None of the companies I call, even the one with the raccoon logo, will actually remove raccoons. The last number I call is Doug's Wildlife Control. Doug tells me that it's now illegal to relocate raccoons but that their arrival is a sign money will come into my life and cayenne won't deter raccoons because it's like Doritos to them and UFOs abduct raccoons rather than any other of Earth's mammals because of their little brain-fingers and did I personally know Susan Sarandon whose name is also Susan (see 41. Individuation) and also people are too paranoid because he has scooped raccoon scat with his bare hands with no ill effects.

I move on to researching deterrents and, after many sunny mornings of expectation turned exasperation at the sight of fresh seedy coils on the gravel, I triumph. You are about to read what may be the only useful information in this book, so listen up. When trying to deter an animal, research the various methods and then Do All Of Them. Three tubes' worth of tennis balls soaked in ammonia are only mildly off-putting. Thorny rose branches alone can be stepped around. Kitty litter clumps alone merely bemuse. Flashing lights alone open a poop disco. Cayenne = Doritos.

But in concert, all this nonsense convinces raccoons their favourite bathroom no longer provides the sanctuary it once did.

I use the same combined-arms approach when two mice saunter past the couch and perform two teensy double-takes, incredulous that I sit on their preferred sofa. Did you know that mice can carry hantavirus which, though rare, boasts a 38 percent mortality rate? The things to do: tuck dryer sheets hither and thither (they find these repellant – and after handling many of them I myself develop weird bumps on the inside of my mouth, though that could be either the hantavirus or menopause), populate your outlets with ultrasonic plug-ins, scour behind and under things you've never even looked behind or under, remove leftover Easter chocolate from the piano bench, sweep leftover Christmas-stocking chocolate from beneath the bed, dig leftover Halloween chocolate from among the Calico Critters in the Calico Critters Caravan Family Camper. Dispose of all leftover sacred and profane chocolate. I've heard that peppermint offends mice, but judging by the interminable baseboard trails of silver-and-red foil scraps punctuated by white-and-red Hershey's CANDY CANE banners, it's like Doritos to them.

And most importantly, set live traps. Every night I plate some almond butter in an enticing manner (dollop and swoop looks good) on the floor of the metal trap and close the lid. By dawn I awaken to tinny thwicks, lift the now marginally heavier trap to peer through the slats at a whiskery silhouette, and chauffeur the mouse-in-a-box to an appealing habitat far enough away that it won't Incredible

Journey back to my piano bench. One evening I hear the thwicks close to midnight and know I will have to drive out to a deserted concession road in the dark, trusting my headlights to confirm that the mouse has indeed scurried out of the trap, hoping no perv happens by while I, spotlit, liberate my little friend by a boggy ditch plumed with invasive phragmites. The problem is mice don't always leap from the trap, as you might expect. Either they don't wish to abandon the rink of almond butter they just perfected a camel spin on or fear has stunned them. We both have to muster a little courage tonight; personally, I channel my mother who, while the size of a mouse herself, fears nothing in the natural world. If I could choose my death from a dropdown menu, I would select 'In my sleep,' duh; she would click 'Other' and write in 'Mauled by lion or grizzly. Shark okay.'

My sense of doing the right thing cancels out the mild heebie-jeebieness of this escapade. My guests will suffer neither poison nor cruel snap-trap deaths. While mouse-deterrent googling, however, I make the mistake of reading what PETA has to say. PETA informs me that live-trapping and releasing breaks up mouse families, causing stress. I brake for squirrels and carry spiders out of the house on folded midterm exams and rescue mayflies from the spider-webs probably spun by those very spiders. But I'm drawing the line here. What do you want from me, PETA?! Shall I leave the exponentially reproductive clan of constantly turding rodents be? Make loveseats for them out of organic strawberries? Will they then eat their own furniture, nibbling around the green calyx stars they proceed to wear as darling hats, but I won't take photos because animals are not here for our entertainment, PETA?!

And I'm sorry, but the ants, the *formica* in formication, they have to go. No humane traps or midterm rides for these guys. Would I feel different if they were a thousand times bigger, if I could see myselves in those compound eyes or admire the way they gingerly suspend a basketball-sized blob of honeydew between tree-saw mandibles? If they wore eyelet lace-trimmed dresses like the Calico Critter mice? Maybe. All I know is I can feel them between my toes right now.

20. URINARY INCONTINENCE

Remember when you were a kid and nirvana lay in pastel candy shaped like garbage (an old shoe! a tin can! ribby little fish carcasses!) packaged in mini garbage pails of vivid colours that snapped open and shut as smartly as a locket and that you could repurpose (pebble keepers, bead stashes, lost-tooth bins, actual garbage pails for Troll dolls) and you went to the dentist and got half your mouth frozen, and they told you not to eat for two hours so you thought well, I'll just have a pail of grape juice then, and stood by the fridge, lifted the still-candy-scented shamrock-green pail to your lips and it was like your mouth forgot what to do because the juice just washed and glubbered down your chin to the floor?

It's like that.

It's happened to me twice so far. The first time, I was driving a few hours up the highway to do a poetry reading at a university, and found myself very very late. The highway was one inexorable gauntlet of safety cones and parked excavators and indecipherable lane markers and flashing 4 km/h speed limits. No time to stop for food, so I compensated by hydrating from my voluminous thermos as I drove. No time for bathroom breaks.

Entering the confounding Venn diagrams of Kitchener and Waterloo, I didn't know exactly where I was going, entirely dependent on the map in my phone. Distracted by the clock, which counted forwards as eagerly as I had once counted backwards (see 35. Itching), I almost rear-ended a bus, kicked the brake, and my phone sailed to the floor. I drove wantonly, hoping for a red light now so I could retrieve my navigator. The reading was meant to have started ten minutes ago. It was a Friday afternoon. No doubt students slumped in a fluorescent-lit classroom, checking their own phones, utterly confident of their co-ordinates and looking forward to escaping them.

Red light. I lunged for my phone, folding myself over the seatbelt. And evidently folding the water balloon inside of me. A water balloon with a knot looser than it used to be.

So now I had not only to locate the venue, but find a bathroom as well, so I could deal with the piss mess before standing at the front of a classroom to share my delightful poems.

When I arrived at the reading, nerves flailing, blazer arms tied around my waist, the organizers commiserated about highway construction and confusing campus layouts, but I could tell the young folk suspected I might be a diva, heedless of their Friday evening plans.

Yet they did not suspect the truth, which I never told, because I hadn't made it to the 45. Fewer Shits stage. Now I might say 'Sorry, you guys! Apparently I pee my pants now. I just chucked my favourite pair of Jockeys out in Philosophy!'

The second time (by the way, I'm feeling pretty good about this book landing me a date), I lazed on a beach thronged with tropical bikinis wearing the black head-to-toe UV suit that protects my vitiligo from the sun (again, confident about those dates), and I was putting off visiting the dank cement bathrooms, which would involve peeling off the damp black suit and swimsuit underneath it. You might say, Why not go in the ocean? But while I will pee in a Northern Ontario cottage lake – sorry, Mum! – I couldn't do it here, in the jewelly coral reef I snorkel thanks to Hawaiian cousins. It feels okay to urinate into cold murky lakes full of Jurassic snapping turtles and bladderwort, but I just can't do it to those E.T.-eyed honu drifting through crystalline robin's-egg waters.

Again, it was the folding. From a prone position I crunched up swiftly to catch a trade wind–blown Funyuns bag and suffered another grape juice incident. It wicked down my wetsuit invisibly, however, so no one ever need know. Except all y'all, I guess.

I've been Kegeling it up. A Kegel sounds like a noodle casserole but is actually a nether-zone exercise that's imperceptible to an outside observer. It can make you feel squeamish at first, that sensation of a vacuum hose sucking up half a sock. It might look like I'm just googling lake plants at my desk, but I'm also knotting a cherry stem inside my mouth and tying a balloon betwixt my hips.

If, despite the Kegels and avoidance of full-bladder acrobatics, urinary incontinence starts happening on the regular, I will be getting some of those new absorbent underwear that I wish had been invented earlier (see 3. Cessation of Menses). They are surprisingly adorable. I've never understood why so many accoutrements for the aging, like orthopedic shoes, come in only two colours: snail and dead snail. Tropical bikinis, brilliant as garbage pails, for me and my peers!

21. ANXIETY[1]

1. See 11. Anxiety.

22. TINNITUS

Tinnnnnnnnnnnnnnnnnnnnnnnnnnnnnnnnnnnnnnnnnnnnnnnnnnnnnnnnnnnnnnnnnnn
nnnnnnnnnnnnnnnnnnnnnnnnnnnnnnnnnnnnnnnnnnnnnnnnnnnnnnnnnnnnnnnnnnnnn
nnnnnnnnnnnnnnnnnnnnnnnnnnnnnnnnnnnnnnnnnnnnnnnnnnnnnnnnnnnnnnnnnnnnn
nnnnnnnnnnnnnnnnnnnnnnnnnnnnnnnnnnnnnnnnnnnnnnnnnnnnnnnnnnnnnnnnnnnnn
nnnnnnnnnnnnnnnnnnnnnnnnnnnnnnnnnnnnnnnnnnnnnnnnnnnnnnnnnnnnnnnnnnnnn
nnnnnnnnnnnnnnnnnnnnnnnnnnnnnnnnnnnnnnnnnnnnnnnnnnnnnnnnnnnnnnnnnnnnn
nnnnnnnnnnnnnnnnnnnnnnnnnnnnnnnnnnnnnnnnnnnnnnnnnnnnnnnnnnnnnnnnnnnnn
nnnnnnnnnnnnnnnnnnnnnnnnnnnnnnnnnnnnnnnnnnnnnnnnnnnnnnnnnnnnnnnnnnnnn
nnnnnnnnnnnnnnnnnnnnnnnnnnnnnnnnnnnnnnnnnnnnnnnnnnnnnnnnnnnnnnnnnnnnn
nnnnnnnnnnnnnnitinsistsnnnnnnnnnnnnnnnnnnnnnnnnnnnnnnnnnnnnnnnnnnnnnn
nnnnnnnnnnnnnnnnnnnnnnnnnnnnnnnnnnnnnnnnnnnnnnnnnnnnnnnnnnnnnnnnnnnnn
nnnnnnnnnn ~~We had a big book called the The Human Body~~ nnnnnnnnnnnn
nnnnnnnnnn ~~when I was a child, full of jaunty anatomies and~~ nnnnnnnnn
nnnnnnnnnn ~~laychild's explanations of physiology. Little men~~ nnnnnnnnn
nnnnnnnnnn ~~in hard hats getting shit done inside me.~~ nnnnnnnnnnnnnnn
nnnnnnnnnnnnnnnnnnnnnnnnnnnnnnnnnnnnnnnnnnnnnnnnnnnnnnnnnnnnnnnnnnnnn
nnnnnnnnnn ~~So I know that in my ear labours a diminutive~~ nnnnnnnnnnn
nnnnnnnitstu ~~piano tuner, knocking various forks against his~~ nnnnnnnnn
nnnnnnnnnn ~~hard hat, sussing out which produces the most~~ nnnnnnnnnnn
nnnnnnnnnn ~~penetrating ring. It is also possible a brood of~~ nnnnnnnnnn
nnnnnnnnnn ~~cicadas shivers their cymbals in here. Either way,~~ nnnnnnnn
nnnnnnnnnisitsi ~~I can't hear you.~~ nnnnnnnnnnnnnnnnnnnnnnnnnnnnnnnnnn
nnnnnnnnnnnnnnnnnnnnnnnnnnnnnnnnnnnnnnnnnnnnnnnnnnnnnnnnnnnnnnnnnnnnn
nnnnnnnnnnnnnnnnnnnnnnnnnnnnnnnnnnnnnnnnnnnnnnnnnnnnnnnnnnnnnnnnnnnnn
nnnnnnnnnnnnnnnnnnnnnnnnnnnnnnnnnnnnnnnnnnnnnnnnnnnnnnnnnnnnnnnnnnnnn
nnnnnnnnnnnnnnnnnnnnnnnnnnnnnnnnnnnnnit'snutsnnnnnnnnnnnnnnnnnnnnnnnn
nnnnnnnnnnnnnnnnnnnnnnnnnnnnnnnnnnnnnnnnnnnnnnnnnnnnnnnnnnnnnnnnnnnnn
nnnnnnnnnnnnnnnnnnnnnnnnnnnnnnnnnnnnnnnnnnnnnnnnnnnnnnnnnnnnnnnnnnnnn
nnnnnnnnnnnnnnnnnnnnnnnnnnnnnnnnnnnnnnnnnnnnnnnnnnnnnnnnnnnnnnnnnnnnn
nnnnnnnnnnnnnnnnnnnnnnnnnnnnnnnnnnnnnnnnnnnnnnnnnnnnnnnnnnnnnnnnnnnnn
nnnnnnnnnnnnnnnnnnnnnnnnnnnnnnnnnnnnnnnnnnnnnnnnnnnnnnnnnnnnnnnnnnnnn
nnntuttiintutusnnnnnnnnnnnnnnnnnnnnnnnnnnnnnnnnnnnnnnnnnnnnnnnnnnnnnn
nnnnnnnnnnnnnnnnnnnnnnnnnnnnnnnnnnnnnnnnnnnnnnnnnnnnnnnnnnnnnnnnnnnnn
nnnnnnnnnnnnnnnnnnnnnnnnnnnnnnnnnnnnnnnnnnnnnnnnnnnnnnnnnnnnnnnnnnnnn
nnnnnnnnnnnnnnnnnnnnnnnnnnnnnnnnnnnnnnnnnnnnnnnnnnnnnnnnnnnnnnnnnnnnn
nnnnnnnnnnnnnnnnnnnnnnnnnnnnnnnit'stitsinnit?nnnnnnnnnnnnnnnnnnnnnnnn
nnnnnnnnnnnnnnnnnnnnnnnnnnnnnnnnnnnnnnnnnnnnnnnnnnnnnnnnnnnnnnnnnnnnn
nnnnnnnnnnnnnnnnnnnnnnnnnnnnnnnnnnnnnnnnnnnnnnnnnnnnnnnnnnnnnnnnnnitus

23. THINNING HAIR

You say that like it's a bad thing. After decades of chomping away at my yak-pelt mop with thinning shears, all I can say is thank god.

According to my hairdresser, when folks hit middle age, men's hair migrates from their scalps down to their backs, and women's hair migrates from their scalps down to their chins. If *Macbeth*'s Banquo had studied cosmetology he wouldn't have been so confused by the three witches, complaining, 'You should be women, and yet your beards forbid me to interpret that you are so.'

I don't have chin hairs yet, but my locks are on their way down. The other day I was brushing my bangs out of my eyes and one hair wouldn't budge. One very fine platinum strand, glued. I tugged at it. One very *long* fine Barbie-platinum strand that, when pulled, pitched a tiny skin-tent in the middle of my forehead. How could this have been here, emerging from the third eye–region of my brow, long enough to grow four inches unnoticed? Did I extrude it overnight?

I guess the only logical conclusion to draw is that I am going through The Change and will soon be a unicorn. My dense thatch of hair will wave out rose gold and aquamarine and my feet will harden into glistering hooves.

But let's get real. I am not becoming a unicorn; I am becoming a narwhal. Because a narwhal is a real thing. Most probably you know that. And I hereby admit to you that I did not always know. I believed narwhals were fantastical until I was far too old. Not forehead-hair old, but definitely an adult when I first saw a photograph of narwhals poking their barley-twist tusks out of icy Arctic waters, conducting the air.

It makes so much sense. We both like to swim. We both have mottled pigmentation. We enjoy calamari. We could be killed easily by either a polar bear or human. We have about twenty friends. We sometimes communicate with them through whistles and clicks. We like to mate among the pack ice. And while female narwhals only rarely sprout tusks, they *can*, Banquo.

24. IRRITABILITY

25. FATIGUE

What with the insomnia (see 9. Insomnia), raccoons (see 19. Formication), and art thieving (see 43. Invisibility Cloak), is it any wonder?

'Fatigue.' Such an apt word. Sounds more tired than 'tired.' With fatigue you are so exhausted you can't even pronounce the final two vowels. Because it's French, and everybody knows the French appreciate a nap.

I grew up in a Mediterranean home, at least in that regard. Though our name for it smacks of Brit: Quiet Time. Fifty years later, it finally hits me that my mother instituted Quiet Time to get a break from us. We didn't have to sleep – we could read or depress the levers of our View-Masters gently – but the point was to take a brief hiatus from scream contests and snow shovel–fencing so she could lie down for thirty minutes and put her elbow over her face. To make the reels last longer I'd click languidly through every 3D frame of *Lady and the Tramp*, Grand Canyon National Park, and an urgent gift from our neighbour Mrs. Southworth, *Miracles of Jesus*.

As with many of these symptoms, I'm not convinced my fatigue is any worse now than in my twenties. (Have I been menopausing my whole life?) Though it's foreign behaviour to many of my friends, my sister understands. We can be quite functionally going about our business and then, like wind-up toys (let's say space shuttle and narwhal), our springs lose their torsion, tick tick tick … tick …… tick. If we are home visiting our parents, there's no need to explain before we shuffle off in search of couches, nose cone and tusk drooping. The only difference these days is that now my parents aren't sleeping: they quietly figure sudokus while my sister and I put our elbows over our faces and go torpid.

Given how sleepy I am by nature, I'm not sure how I've done what I've done in life. Not sure how I will finish writing this book. Not even sure if I can wade through

🐑 Pause for Quiet Time, or, Jesus Casts out Demons into Pigs 🐑

this paragraph. How have famous artists and thinkers managed to produce so much? I know, mostly thanks to Mason Currey's lovely exploration of creative routines, *Daily Rituals: How Artists Work*, that there are some things I could try. Like W. H. Auden, Graham Greene, and Jean-Paul Sartre, I could take amphetamines. Cocaine seemed to help Sigmund Freud and Thomas Edison, who didn't understand why nobody else could work for seventy-two hours straight. For most of the greats, the massive quantities of coffee, cigarettes, cigars, and pipes baffle measure. Though if you do want to measure, Balzac drank upwards of fifty cups of coffee daily, and Freud smoked twenty cigars a day.

The other must for anyone wishing to devote their limited energies to creative work is to have a wife and/or servants do absolutely everything for you. You can even have children without ever taking care of them! Back to Freud – why is he always at the ready to leap out of my unconscious? – whose wife laid his clothes out for him and applied toothpaste to his toothbrush. Mahler's young wife kept things silent for the composer, including refraining from playing the piano and, at his insistence, giving up her own career as a composer. Unsurprisingly, we find only a few of the female greats had a share of this benefit: Jane Austen's sister Cassandra took on Jane's housework duties and Gertrude Stein's devoted wife, Alice, shielded the genius from all domestic chores.

I don't have a wife, cigars, or even coffee, and the only bennies I take involve poached eggs. But there's another thing creative greats have done, and that's take naps. (This includes the sleep-shaming Edison, who in truth popped off for siestas; perhaps his brief, intensive conk-outs on a lab bench or pile of pipes reveal not his ruggedness but his exhaustion.) I will work tirelessly to emulate the nappers.

I find myself wondering if 'Quiet Time' exists outside our home, and my research reveals that I'm supposed to devote it to adoring, beholding, and praying to God. Mrs. Southworth, it all makes sense now! It's also a term for toddler rests, so if you can't yet pick out your own outfits or brush your own teeth, it might be for you.

26. PALPITATIONS

They go boopa boopa boopap .... Kathunka! boopap boop boop .... bip Kathwapp!

These are palpitations. As in, palpable weird heartbeats. I can feel them flip inside me, hear them as intermittent hail on a tin roof, some pea-sized, some tennis ball. You can see them, boopap-ing out, a valentine chocolate box straining against the skin of my chest.

I am surrounded by 'doctors' at work, who suggest there are spondees in my trochees, that my rhythm has sprung. Dr. Matheson whispers that my corset might be too tight.

So I go to my real doctor, who whips out his stethoscope and listens for a while, humouring me.

'Well, it's probably nothing to worry about.'

Probably? (See 11. Anxiety.)

He comforts and edifies me: 'It's a rhythmic arrhythmia.' I think I am supposed to chuckle at the oxymoron, as at 'jumbo shrimp' or 'creative nonfiction.' He's becoming accustomed to my anxious queries. The truth is, he doesn't say but implies with a wry half-smile born of uneven cheek Botox, that the diagnosis for most of my bodily failings is aging. There's nothing to be done about it. And then when your heart stops beating and you collapse, pale and breathless, it's still nothing to worry about. You're just dead.

27. CHANGES IN TASTE

Before Meno.	After Meno.
- Milk choc. easter bunny (+xtra eyes)	- Cacao Nibs (eyes mixed in) BulkBarn
- Staying out of it	- telling everybody what's what
- Doc Ms	- orthotics (in Doc MS)
- chaos	- columns
- 8 cats	- 2 cats
- mushrooms NO	- mushrooms YES
- low femme plaid granola boho	- onesie
- strings	- horns
- parsnips No	- parsnips yes still NO
- sorry	- Not sorry
- leg shaving	- log shoving
- dance like nobody's watching	- dance like everbody's watching + wants lessons from me
- Red Bull	- Pitbull
- answering questions with questions	- questioning answers with answers
- caretaking	- Naps
- mentoring	- ice cream sandwiches (Neop-litan), strawberry end 1st

28. SWARMING OF ENTRAILS

Kidding. That doesn't appear on any contemporary list. But don't dismiss tradition. In addition to hot flashes and fatigue, watch out for involuntary laughing, an impulse to steal, scurvy, bleeding from the ears, Satan lodging in your hipbones, and 'Regurgitation, at length, of the uterine milk into the blood.' Check, check, check, check, check, and check!

What did 'swarming of entrails' actually mean? Butterflies in the stomach, an aspect of the 'intense sexual ardour' Andrew Currier warned of in his 1897 book on menopause? Age-related lactose intolerance? Have my entrails ever swarmed? I feel like they have. Maybe a few hours after a boss's party where I bit into a piece of Jello-y under-barbecued chicken that I was too polite and precariously employed to spit out.

I'm stumped by the term 'entrails,' which I never imagine housed in a living body. Entrails are what slide out when a lion tears open the belly of a kill. A haruspex tosses entrails on the temple floor to portend fortunes. Intestines, bowels: these still work. Even the coils of slimy bratwurst Dr. Miranda Bailey probes and juggles in the O.R. are still intestines to me, as long as the patient lives. After the flat-line ohmmmms and she concedes a time of death, it's entrails she tucks back in and sews shut.

Wait until I'm dead to read my entrails. If you rip them out when they are still swarming and divine that my death is nigh, that's a bit of a cheat.

29. DRY EYES

L

The audience watches the scene where the dog dies and there *is* a dry eye in the place. It's mine! Not because I am a cat person and/or cold-hearted. For most of my life you could count on me to descend into blubbery convulsions at a filmic dog death or an airport farewell or, of course, a real dog death. I would readily cry for sad or happy reasons any old time. Now you can rarely squeeze a sob out of me. Maybe I've used up all my tears along with my eggs.

Last August, Lori and I left our daughter at university, a nine-hour drive away. Yes, I know that forty pages ago Elise was still in high school, but that tortoise in a baseball cap from 18. Dizzy Spells could serve as my author photo. As we said our

R

When Kelly joined our fifth-grade class mid-year, cliques had already formed. The only way to make her mark was to perform eye tricks on demand: flipping her eyelids inside out, which yielded a kind of zombie-slash-wounded-centipede effect, and touching the white of her eyeball with her finger. Thank goodness I didn't have to cultivate these skills, due to my own negative-attention magnets, mismatched body parts and dorky pants (see 45. Fewer Shits).

I thought of Kelly when my vanity compelled me to change from glasses to contact lenses in my mid-teens. Clearly it was possible to touch your eye. But you bring that glassy little saucer, stuck to your index finger, toward your iris, and every goodbyes, she and her other mom bawled unabashedly on the Montréal sidewalk while I comforted them, stoic as a 1950s dad. But then, I had been preparing for this for months, years even, so it's not like Elise leaving was a surprise. She walked toward her residence building and I settled into the car with a bag of warm all-dressed bagels on my lap. But before Lori could turn on the ignition I blurted, 'Give me a minute.' I covered my face with my hands and hunched over, crushing the bagel bag, which ripped and slipped to the floor and down fell my newborn with the lavender milk head, down fell the wonder-eyed baby poking spitty fingers into my mouth, down fell my cheeky toddler bringing me a dozenth book to read. Lori gathered my motormouth little kindergartner off the

instinct compels you to snap your lids shut. My eye was an open window to a proverbial soul quivering inside. I scrunched my lids onto the contact over and over until my face grew red and wet and the lens had been folded and inverted so many times the optometrist stopped assuring me the eye is a rubber ball and suggested I try again tomorrow. So many things are like learning to ride a bicycle, and inserting a contact lens is one of them; when you can't do it, you can't do it, and then when you can, you can.

I'm back to glasses now but recently popped in some contacts for swimming reasons. When I got home, I discovered I could not get them out. I pinched and pinched at my eyeballs over the bathroom sink, totally putting Kelly to shame, but found it impossible to get any purchase. If I couldn't see floor mat and tossed her into the back seat and gone was my chortle-buddy playing Rhyme Out way past bedtime, gone my tween who still linked arms with me at the grocery store, gone the young woman who became my BFF, thousands upon thousands of glitter-lit days all wrenched away from me at once, cradle and all, and crashing out of me came what I can only describe as bull-elk bugling. Not because she heard this, but because she turned back for one more hug, Elise appeared at my window. At least she knew I was feeling a feeling about saying goodbye.

Between you and me, the next time I cried after that was right now, writing this. Which makes me laugh (see 5. Mood Swings™).

individual hornets papping the sappy pears outside my window so well I would never have believed the contacts were still in there. There had to be some hack for this, some secret trick. I got a little panicky and sought out the book perched on the edge of the bathtub, a moist medieval treatise called *De Secretis Mulierum (Women's Secrets)*, which told me that because I no longer menstruate, I could poison the eyes of a babe in the cradle just by looking at it. I googled the issue, scanning phrases (blurred because my contacts correct myopia rather than hyperopia) for a remedy. No, my phone is not stuck in Contacts. No, I don't need contact cement. Finally, I read that all I need to do is pour some saline solution into my eyes and, as it happens, all over my face for a couple of minutes, because that soul-protection instinct dies hard.

30. PANIC DISORDER

Imagine an esteemed medical professional attaching leeches to your vulva. If you don't have a vulva, imagine you have a vulva, and then imagine the leeches. (If you don't have a vulva and you are still reading this book, you get an honorary one.)

In the eighteenth and nineteenth centuries, leeching was a popular treatment for nervous disorders, especially 'climacteric insanity,' that particular brand of crazy that arises when society can't figure out what you're for anymore. Bloodletting follows from the notion held in Classical times that when menstruation ceases, the blood has nowhere to go and starts accumulating in you and wreaking havoc. Makes sense.

I arrive with trepidation at this chapter – in fact, I am composing it last. Because this is getting real. Last year I developed panic attacks and generalized anxiety disorder (don't see 46. Anxiety). The after-effects of concussion (see 18. Dizzy Spells), pandemic hyper-vigilance, new stressors at work and home, and climacteric recalibrations conspired to bring on my first serious mental illness.

It's difficult to explain to the uninitiated. Well-meaning friends suggested exposure therapy: for fear of heights take one step up the ladder, acclimate to that, then another step up, acclimate, up again, etc., until voilà, you are cleaning the eavestroughs. But generalized anxiety disorder is not about fear of something; it's about fear of everything. Every moment spins out on the ice. The steering wheel becomes a feeble toy, and you don't know yet if you will land on the shoulder, in the ditch, or crumpled against the grill of a truck. I remember starting a day that would involve two meetings and five hours of university lecturing, not feeling concerned about those at all but struggling to make Elise's lunch, my thoughts raging, *Can I make this lunch Is it healthy enough Is it enough Can I cut this pepper Can I walk over to the drawer to get the knife Can I hide my mind until she leaves for school?*

I didn't understand, before diagnosis, why I would frequently experience a sudden rising dread, a near faint, an instinctive and desperate struggle to conceal the adrenaline hurricane surging through my body. One day I was sitting in my parked car, talking on the phone, when the leviathan began to loom. I lost my ability to enunciate for the violent trembling, my heart threatened to seize, frantic wasps dredged my hands and feet. Luckily it was Lori on the phone, who, as a professional counsellor, tried to get me to breathe and assured me I would not die. She asked if I wanted an ambulance. I did and I did not. Many years ago I nearly drowned, ensnared by an urgent current moving beneath the deceptively gentle chipchop surface of the cottage lake. My boyfriend Kevin stood up on the dock, wondering why I didn't advance. I thought of raising my arm for help, but knew the minute I did so, I'd be admitting to myself the peril I was in, and the act of surrender would drown me. I had the same feeling about calling an ambulance. So Lori called Dr. Matheson, who had to leave a yoga class to drive around searching for my car, where she sat with me quietly while my breath slowed, then assured me that spontaneous overflows of powerful feelings are normal, and that one day I would recollect them in tranquillity and maybe write about them.

That day I realized I could not handle the panic episodes on my own, and needed to talk to my doctor about medication. I would tread water in the vortex for a minute and raise my arm.

A year later my heart dances with the daffodils. I found a drug that muffles my panic but not my joy. It can take a few attempts, however, to identify the prescription that works for you. Third try was a charm, but first I had to endure one pill that decimated my white blood cell count, and then there were the leeches, which just gave me more panic attacks.

31. METALLIC TASTE IN THE MOUTH

Pins. Needles. Keys. Nails. Paper clips. Cutlery. Every day, so probably around 60,000 pieces of cutlery. My tongue loves being little-spooned and tine-runnelled. Flask. Someone else's braces. Coins. If I had more than fifty-three in my leopard piggy bank I might have gone for the world record (now 411, by Dinesh Shivnath Upadhyaya in 2015). Frozen pole. Does foil count? Someone else's zipper. The end of a small flashlight, while replacing the furnace filter in a webby crawl space. The other end of a big flashlight, bulbed cheeks a flamingo neon in the tent, as dark sleet pummelled the tarp like a million ball bearings seeking a mouth.

32. LOSS OF MUSCLE MASS

Joke's on you, menopause. I never had any to begin with!

33. REDUCED LIBIDO

I'm tempted to evade the above topic by discussing at length the etymology of *libido*, purportedly from the Latin, though possibly of Minion origin. Can I write a memoir about menopause if I keep getting bashful about the personal? Wait, do Minions have libidos?

a) No
b) As with humans, there's great variation in the sexual ideation and responsiveness of Minions
c) In spades
d) What are you picturing right now?
e) Don't answer that.

In other words, at times I embark on a chapter and worry, *What would Grandpa think?!* My father's father's first name, Leslie, is my middle. He was too loud and I loved it. He would always hammer out 'Oh! Susannah' on the piano for me. When at five I peed the bed (see 20. Urinary Incontinence), he changed the sheets and remarked on how wily rain can be, twisting through the window screen like that. He made extra sure to treat me like the cheese after my adorable eleven-years-younger twin siblings were born. But he had also trained in Anglican theology and became uncharacteristically silent when encountering the futon I shared with Kevin during undergrad, as if he had expected to find separate bedrooms in our one-bedroom apartment.

Around that time, I watched *50 Weeks* or *9½ Shades of Grey* or whatever it's called. The only thing that stayed with me was a scene where curator Kim Basinger visits the artist Farnsworth, an elderly man who inhabits a cottage in the sun-dappled countryside. She has been embroiled in a toxic spiral of erotic adventures with Mickey Rourke (character name John *Gray*!), and this outing gifts her a serene space, replete with pure creative energy all the more luminous for its remove from the manipulative sexual thrall sapping her. There is also a fish, but I don't know what that's about. Years later I found myself in a toxic-thrall situation, and this scene popped into my head, reminding me that I could escape into a more peaceful kind of joy. Sometimes I fantasized about an angst-free, sexually calmed old age similar to Farnsworth's. I could paint still lives among illumined motes of dust. Maybe menopause would offer that?

Historically, older women have been deemed either 'sexual neuters' (a term found in Dr. Robert A. Wilson's bestseller *Feminine Forever*) or subject to oversexed 'fureur utérine' (uterine furor) (so said Dr. Charles de Gardanne, the man who coined the term 'ménopause'). Which is it, fellas? As with the 'weight gain' symptom (see next chapter), both lived experiences and medical observations are all over the map, with the cultural attitudes and commercial interests of any given era and place often contouring the facts. While after three decades and billions of dollars worth of Viagra, there is some attention turning now to midlife reductions in female libido, in the nineteenth century it was the phenomenon of *increased* menopausal sex drive that prompted hand-wringing among medical men. With her reproductive life over, a woman's erotic desire was considered monstrous and labelled nymphomania. Indulging it could lead to insanity and death, so surgically removing a randy woman's ovaries, womb, and, oh why not, clitoris became a popular cure.

From my grandfather I inherited not only a name but curiosity about aging. He wrote a syndicated column called 'The Fourth Quarter.' When the *Globe and Mail* arrived, ten-year-old me would lay it on the kitchen table next to my Lucky Charms, rattle it open to the Thursday Section (formerly the Women's Section, until women suggested they were capable of reading the entire newspaper), and study what Grandpa had to say about pension management, phased retirement, navigating the medical establishment, husbands peeling potatoes, and how to spot hucksters who target the grey-haired set. I found it a challenge not to get so engrossed that the NEW blue diamonds lost their dry-sponge crunch to the milk. He went on to write a Minion-yellow book called *Improving with Age*, which I shelved by my bed in a place of honour between *Anne of Green Gables* and *Mad Libs*. While I read with interest the chapters on bone density and keeping busy, I stopped cold at the one where the word 'orgasm' appears in the first sentence. For a kid unfamiliar with mid-century slang, the chapter title, 'Doing What Comes Naturally,' did not serve as a sufficient trigger warning. Grandpa?! *Grandma?!?!* I don't recall finishing the chapter but I must have, because flipping through that dusty copy of *Mad Libs* I encountered years later:

A DAY AT THE ZOO

It was a <u>transurethral</u> afternoon.
ADJECTIVE

The <u>nipple</u> cages were <u>expulsive</u> with chattering <u>glands</u> .
    NOUN   ADJECTIVE   PLURAL NOUN

<u>Loins</u> roared in the <u>rectum</u>.
NOUN   NOUN

<u>Masters</u> and <u>Johnson</u> shared a bag of <u>penis</u> with the elephant.
NAME   NAME   NOUN

<u>Swelling</u> in the pond were a <u>love</u> and a <u>orgasm</u>.
VERB   NOUN   NOUN

I guess we're even now, Grandpa.

34. WEIGHT GAIN

After all this talk of losses – libido, muscle mass, fertility, memory, hair – finally a gain! Let's put on our stretchy pants and celebrate!

The Victorian physician George Corfe warns that in menopause 'fat now takes the place of muscles, glands, and even bones.' And I thought I was able to reach into the back seat behind me thanks to double-jointed elbows, when it's really because I have bones of butter.

At the same time, you can find nineteenth-century experts complaining a middle-aged woman becomes less feminine as her 'form becomes angular, the body lean.'

Sounds like it doesn't matter if and how your weight changes during menopause, your body is, as usual, somehow wrong. Whether you gain or lose, you lose.

On average, women gain 1.5 pounds a year during their fifties. That tracks with the anecdotal evidence from my friends and my own belt holes. We have already touched upon the freshman fifteen, acquired when leaving home and adopting a diet of tater tots and vodka coolers. We can call menopausal gain the 'fewer shits fifteen' (see 45. Fewer Shits).

If you were to argue that I don't really know what I'm talking about when it comes to weight issues because both my parents need suspenders to keep their gardening pants up, you'd be right. I don't wish to diminish the experiences of those who have had to struggle to lose weight, but I distrust the culture of body surveillance that encourages shame and anxiety about it, and about the common upsize or two in midlife.

You'd think the world has a problem with women taking up more space.

35. ITCHING

Lifetime Top Five countdown:

5. My older brother Michael got the chicken pox at eight, so I was just a tot when I caught it, but became well versed in the spectre of oozing infections and hideous scars should I scratch the blossoming polka dots. An obedient child, I sat very still in my room, sequined with calamine. Despite my desperate desire to tear around scraping myself against every chair and doorframe in the house, I budged only to take a quick call on my pull-along Chatter Telephone. With my pink-spotted foot, I drove it forward and back on the floor, goading its rolling eyes into a frenzy.

4. My family moved back to Canada from California when I was five, and my parents deposited me with my Ottawa cousins while they searched for somewhere to live in Guelph. What a delirious party for me to be left with three girl cousins – two to play with and an older one to worship. Making merry one night, I clambered up my bunk-bed ladder, arms stuffed with stuffies, and then someone squeaked and we all smashed to the floor. Eleanor's trunk was trapped under Ling-Ling. Brownie lost an eye. Woody Woodpecker's pull-string caught on a rung and he dangled, laughing nervously. Uncle Ron (human) ran into the sorry menagerie and tenderly straightened my arm, which made a sound like kindling popping in a fire. Aunt Barbara knotted a paisley bandana sling and we beat it through the dark to the hospital, me

on Barbara's lap in the passenger seat, yellow ribbons of light swimming over our bodies.

All I remember from the emergency room is a bloody man staggering in, slurring, 'My car! My car!' On the operating table, the anaesthetist asked me if I knew how to count backwards. *Do I know how to count backwards? Dude, watch and learn.* A second later I woke up in sunlit sheets, with an L-shaped cast on my arm. Sometime between 'My car!' and 'One hundred, ninety-nine, ninety-eight, ninety-shuuhhh … ' police hustled to locate my parents, calling every motel in Guelph in search of the go-ahead for an operation. At last, at 2 a.m., they got my parents' room at the Parkview. My father picked up the phone in the black and heard 'This is the Ontario Provincial Police. Your daughter's been in a serious accident and we need your permission to perform emergency surgery.' The story goes that my intellectually commanding, unflappable, and eminently capable father handed the phone to my mother. They drove the six hours to Ottawa imagining car crashes, snapped spines, slurring bloody men. When they arrived, the orthopedic surgeon told my mother, sombrely, that I'd broken my elbow falling off a bunk bed. She appalled him with her gleeful 'Oh is that *all*?!'

That's the short story long that led to my cast itch. Now that playgrounds are designed to keep children intact – no more sliding down hot razors, no more getting bludgeoned by petrified tractor tires – you hardly ever see a kid in a cast. In my day we were forever doodling Muppets and *Grease* lyrics on the plaster limbs of our classmates. But if you've had a cast, you know that special breed of itch, the kind you literally cannot scratch. Brushy-legged bugs zinging around in there (see 19. Formication), French-braiding your arm hairs, signing your actual arm, tickling out the lyrics to 'There Are Worse Things I Could Do.'

3. According to my research, *Candida* is either a unique fusion of opera and musical theatre that features 'irreverence' and 'biting humour' or the twenty-fifth greatest play of all time, which 'bristles with Shavian wit.' This explains the bristling, biting, and irreverence I suffered in my late twenties. When you become chronically overwhelmed or anxious, your cortisol levels rise, which in turn leads to the excess blood sugar that promotes yeast growth. Because what you need when you already have more on your plate than you can handle is a wad of expanding dough flumped on top of it all.

Most people with vaginas will get at least one yeast infection in their lives. But you will not see these people scratching themselves in public, even if their operetta has been agitating the hell out of them with no intermission in sight. Many with twig and berries, on the other hand, scratch away on the bus, in front of the yogurt display, in the airplane seat beside you. Why are you guys so itchy? The more discreet fellows will look off into the distance, because if they can't see you, you can't see them. The question is, do we want to feel free to scratch too or do we want them to stop? Kindly write your answer on the back of your ticket and drop it at the box office on your way out.

2. On every high school boyfriend's wall, Farrah Fawcett bared maybe two complete sets of teeth, her loose ringlets a whorled gilt frame around her California-tan face. Fawcett in her iconic red swimsuit, happy-nippled, the bestselling poster of all time. First day of March Break 1982, Cindy and I were hell-bent on acquiring her golden tan, horsing around in the sun-tossing Florida surf and adhering to our beach towels, this being the era when people coated themselves in coconut oil rather than sunscreen. We achieved the iconic red everywhere but our swimsuits.

Katsuobushi, or Bonito flakes, are tissue-thin fish shavings that shimmy and wave, in a manner both wowing and disturbing, when plated on top of hot food. Twitching and squirming on a sand-dollar coverlet, dreaming of sleep, I could swear my sunburn was doing that. As hot food cools, Bonito flakes slow and still. But my body was not a cooling dish. I blazed incessantly, skin peeling up and doing the worm to 'California Girls' all night long.

P.S. Despite the high school boyfriends with their Farrah Fawcett posters (or because of them?), both Cindy and I ended up gay! (See 'hell-bent' above.)

1. I set my baby on a flannel blanket in the grass and got down to business pulling weeds. Dandelions, fleabane, henbit. And where had all these creeping vines come from? How satisfying to anchor them around my glove and yank, trailing them across my bare legs into a springy pile. I had never encountered these before. The leaves grew in charming compound formation, three leaflets with soft teeth.

Alarm torqued the normally serene voice of the angel on my shoulder: 'Leaves of three, let them be.' While I generally listened to my devil, who was chanting 'Yank! Yank! Yank!,' I paused. As a new mother I had become absurdly overcautious, and felt 95 percent sure I was acting out of the paranoia that, while keeping our species alive for hundreds of millennia, could overshoot the mark. Nevertheless I abandoned operations, rinsed my hands under the hose, and took Elise in for a bath, in case any trace of ivy spittle had landed on her. I have since learned that only one nanogram (a billionth of a gram) of urushiol oil need brush your skin to provoke a rash.

The baby was fine. My legs, on the other hand, teemed with nanograms, bubbling up into blistery welts the itch of which only fellow botanical idiots can understand.

The worst part is that any soothing balm you apply lasts twenty minutes tops, and then you re-hurtle yourself naked-legged toward the cortisone or calamine or Vicks VapoRub or cucumber slurry or shoe polish or combination of all these.

No, the worst part is that if you scratch the itch, it burns like shingles (which feels like being whipped with barbed wire, so get your vaccine![2]). And while objectively poison ivy lasts on average three weeks, subjectively – *this* is the worst part – it lasts a kazillion years.

So, whisking my brittle nails (see ?. Brittle Nails, if I ever write that one) over a funny new tinglebuzz on my forearm

---

2. Shingles arises when the chicken pox virus holing up in your nervous system reactivates. Thanks again, Michael!

is no big deal. Even, like brittle nails, not worth writing home about.

P.S. I wrote that arrogant coda yesterday, and of course last night I was repeatedly awakened by itchy ankles, neck, wrists. Neither Leo nor I can reach the zone between our shoulder blades and must resort to kicking at our ears with our back feet. So scratch that bit.

But don't be too vigorous about it or you'll crack a talon.

36. DRY MOUTH

I feel like my childhood doll Brenda (see 1. Loss of Fertility), in that whatever I tip into my thirsty liphole disappears immediately, down a plastic tube and out another hole between my swivellable legs.

But my driest mouth emerged at a pretty non-menopausal moment, while working my ass off (I'm going to go ahead and say *literally* here, to emphasize the unmistakable feeling that parts of my ass did indeed come off) for twenty-four hours birthing a baby. You are not allowed to eat or drink during labour, in case you require an emergency Caesarean.

This was okay for the first twenty hours, but then I hit the pushing stage, which is when, already utterly spent, you dig the deepest you ever have for the last fraying fibre of push you didn't even know you had, and labour with Olympic powerlifting face while people shout at you. Every couple of minutes they yell, 'Six five four three two one!' and then, cruelly, 'Six five four three two one!' And then again and again and again, as if you won't realize that makes thirty! The charade goes on for about three or forty-five hours. I imagine this is what the final miles of a marathon are like. A marathon with a nebulous finish line. A marathon with a whooping crowd refusing to hand you water. A marathon with someone else's head lodged in your vagina.

I thought back to the 'discomfort' of having to guzzle 1.5 litres of water before an ultrasound or chugging my overfull jug of peppermint tea in the airport security line.

I wanted to go back in time and slap my own face, teach myself something about gratitude, and then slurp up the cheekslosh dislodged by the slapping.

While you may not drink anything during labour, you may dig through ice chips in a styrofoam cup. Here's where a doula's expertise kicks in. Forget the calming voice, capable hands, feminist advocacy, pool noodles, and wisdom of the ages. Doulas slip a shot glass of Sprite into the opaque cup of ice whenever the doctor is either out of the room or engaged in counting centimetres inside you.

Before that day, I had enjoyed the odd root beer or Diet Coke, but Sprite was whatever. On that day, Sprite became my lifeblood, my holiest water, my Louis Roederer Cristal Brut 2014. After every bout of attempting to turn myself inside out, I would grunt 'ice!' but what I meant was 'sweet citrus fizz cut with meltwater to yield an ambrosial frolic across the palate which could slake a cracked sandflat into spontaneous meadow.' My sister Alex, fluent in me, brought the styrofoam to my lips every time.

This relentless wheel of shouting, pushing, and 'ice!' waxed into my delirious forever, my new normal. When Lori, whose job it was to have her hand bones crushed by mine, finally said, 'This is it, one more push! Six five four … ' I was like, yeah yeah yeah you guys. But, shockingly, a real live baby came out of me, and I wept ecstatic tears of Sprite.

Everybody and the baby left the room in a flurry, leaving my doctor and me in a buzzy silence while he sewed me up. I think I asked him if he was stitching my actual butt closed and he just laughed, so I asked again with a 'seriously though' and he laughed again, so I guess I made a joke.

Alex returned. She hadn't gone to the NICU with the others – she had hunted down a vending machine, and now psh-pshted open a full, glimmering, blue-green can, as wondrous as Earth seen from space.

37. BLOATING

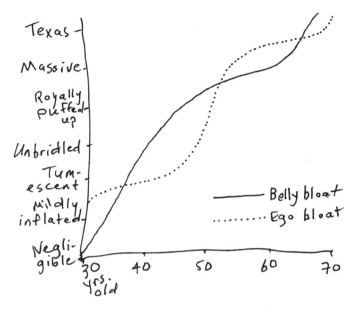

No matter how quickly or slowly I eat or how light or heavy my meals, I always end up feeling full of myself. Sometimes this condition is exacerbated by fluctuating hormones, or an inability to tolerate certain fools. Sometimes it's painful (for other people) or can make you fart (but see 45. Fewer Shits). With menopause I find my bloat is slow to deflate and that's fine. Like the Magnificent Frigatebird (actual species name), I can fly while still ballooning.

38. JOINT PAIN

I need to swallow. *Swallow.* Do I remember how to swallow? What does the tongue do?

When I was a teenager, joints made me giggly. Meeting cloudy pals in a playground at night, having as much fun as we did ten years earlier when we swung and slid and monkeyed. But for a long time since, every time I try cannabis I end up on a paranoia bus I can't get off.

I think I'm meant to do something at the front of the mouth, but also the back. I attempt a constrained rear-door gulp, my go-to at the dentist when they pack my yap with fluoride trays, but can't manage even that. All my friends at this party seem pretty chill even though everybody knows you cannot swallow and breathe at the same time! Pertinent details from Biology class return to me with disquieting clarity. There are a hell of a lot of muscles whose function it is to prevent aspiration and choking. My levator veli palatini, cricoarytenoid, and aryepiglottic muscles await my instructions. What if I cannot accomplish a swallow and I perish, choking on my own saliva? I could spit into my Shiraz but then everyone would know how unchill and gross I am and I would ruin their vibe, which is really good, I can tell, because Susan (see 41. Individuation) and Lindsay (who normally has frozen shoulder[3]) take turns making a cerulean-blue plastic dolphin charm from a Kinder egg perform. It swoops down and swims twist-and-turningly through an imaginary Caribbean sea, then rises to breach

---

3. Another symptom of menopause.

the imaginary gently scalloped surface, executes an end-over-end flip, and they go *Wow*. To my right, Rick breaks Ruffles chips along each pleat with the care of a watchmaker and holds the results between his lips like pins, like a porcupine accident, like a *Hellraiser* demon. That's the only horror movie I ever watched but as with Biology diagrams, some things you can't unsee.

I was so careful this time. I went into a dispensary myself and requested something for a lightweight, a strain that approximates the gentle buzz of a 1985 spliff. 'This will do the trick' they nodded muskily and slipped me a tube of Jinglebell Frolic Creamsicle Hammock.

Come on, swllw. Swllw. My tongue has frozen shoulder. My friends want me to eat the pins. They want me to chew a bear. They do not know I have forgotten how to swallow. Or do they? They may be trying help me form a bolus to kickstart the reflex. They may be trying to kill me.

I would get up but I cannot get up. I forget how. And if I could, I would have to stand there for a few seconds, and I'd be a standing sitting duck. It's my hip. Or, I should say, ma hip, because hips are a seniors' complaint and diphthongs are for the young. Also thongs. If you have hip pain, you know what I'm talking about. If you don't, you've seen it. Maybe in person, when someone gets out of their car and just stands there for a moment before resuming motion, as if stopped in their tracks by the remarkable loveliness of the Pet Valu. They are waiting for their hips to unlock, for the pain to drain out. Or you've seen it in an ibuprofen ad, where a silhouette too athletically shaped for a sufferer nevertheless sports a pulsating sea urchin on his hip. It's red, because that means pain (or Republicans or Valentine's Day – like I said, pain). And it's a scarlet red, the lit-from-within red that distinguishes tanager from cardinal, sour cherry from sweet, flash from blush.

We can blame joint pain on menopause – recall that Satan can inhabit the hipbones at this critical point in a woman's life – but I got my sore hips from my dad who, come to think of it, also gave me 12. Vision Problems, 26. Palpitations, and a horror of horrors.

I'm on the lookout for a remedy. Rick and the internet recommend cannabis.

39. ANXIETY

You will be phone-interviewed by BBC radio at 3 a.m. (agh, time zones) about a book on spirituality you forgot to write.

(See p. 39 of the ninth book from the right on the third shelf of the nearest bookcase, no matter where you are. Find the fifth noun or proper noun (plus descriptor and/or article if present) on that page. This is the title of your book.[4])

(Also see 21. Anxiety.)

---

4. As for me, I will be pulling *The Familiar Brown Jug-worm* out of my ass.

40. DIFFICULTY CONCENTRATING

Declining hormone levels in menopause have been linked to troubles with concentration. Estrogen keeps the neurons firing and regulates glucose transport, aerobic glycolysis, and mitochondrial function. So, with less estrogen, what is the height of Troll dolls? A person can experience cognitive symptoms, because 'any troll at twelve inches or so is considered very large, with trolls over that considered gigantic.' A diet rich in polyunsaturated fatty acids can help support any of that lasagna left? What were ancient Greek pessaries made of? Eggs, fish, nuts, and seeds contain plenty of Omega – Oh meh gah!, at first I thought I would have to eat the dung, but it's more like a suppository. Who ate the lasagna? Garfield places lasagna in his vagina on Mondays. Exercise increases blood flow to the brain, promoting optional performance. Change one letter in Pilates and you get pirates. Let's go to puh-RAH-teez class. Ahrr, anchor that spine! Brave that plank, ye trolls! (See 8. Brain Frog.)

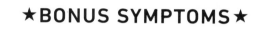

★BONUS SYMPTOMS★

41. INDIVIDUATION

If you didn't know my name and I told you I was writing a book about menopause, you could safely say, 'Interesting. Tell me more, Susan.' You probably wouldn't try 'Interesting, Madysson. Tell me more.'

I already wrote about the phenomenon of the postwar Susan boom for a piece in Sarah Yi-Mei Tsiang's anthology of Canadian poets named Susan, *Desperately Seeking Susans*. But that was 2012. Hi again from all the Susans, who have now gone through The Change. Watch out. Our feet got bigger, we care less about what you think, and you can't swing a cat without hitting one of us, who will then adopt it.

Four of my daughter's best friends have formidable mothers named Susan. To her it's just a synonym for Mom. The remaining moms are Lisas, and you can pretty much throw them in the pot with us.

Paradoxically, the ubiquity of Susan used to make the name indiscernible. You savoured Charmaine, but you swallowed Susan without tasting it. It was like, 'Hello, my name is The.' I envied my friends who were at least given Suzette and Suzanne, the Rosette and Roseanne to my raisin. Yet as we age out of many target demographics and 'become invisible' (see 43. Invisibility Cloak), our name has actually begun to feel almost rare-ish for its now decades-long guttering.

'Susan' tastes pretty. Susan Susan Susan. So curvy you'd think it was cursive. Two different sounds from the same letter, sss zzz. The blanket-rolled ooo vowel and the second syllable's soft landing. Thank you, Catherines and Marys, for giving us such a beautiful name.

This evolution from common sparrow to painted bunting will happen for the Madisons as well. In the retirement home seventy years from now, the nurse will say 'Madisun, time for your pills. No, not you, hon – Madisun in the *red* hoverchair.

'Susan! You *still* here?!'

42. HOTTER FLASHES

Dropping from a dazzled cloudbank, you are the sun's under-boob. You froth over the pasta-pot lip. Bodysurf a velodrome of hot coals. Mile 20 in the Honolulu marathon. You are a VeryBerry bath bomb bleeding apart in the smoking tub. Rolled up in a black plastic tarp, Death Valley asphalt, noon. Trapped on the griddley top bench of an itsy-bitsy sauna because you can't catch an opening to squeeze by the pinking flesh of the contented sighing towelless people who keep getting up to scoop more water onto the scorched rocks, Fttshhhhhhtssss! All four stove coils firing up orange. Three inside your torso and one inside your face. You circumnavigate the globe, doing the worm all along the scarlet equator. In the nursing home, where even the busy staff must move languorously to survive the cranked thermostat, you nestle under an afghan on the velour loveseat, cockblocking a heat-wheezing geezer on your left and your grandma on your right, who's crocheting you another afghan. You are body-snatched into a locked sunbed for the long weekend. You are whatever Jennifer Beals is welding in *Flashdance*. You got your head caught in a hydrothermal vent on the deepest of indifferent seafloors, where extreme shrimp frolic among the toxic 750° jets. You are soup[5]. You are lava. You are quark-gluon plasma.

---

5. Vent-shrimp soup.

43. INVISIBILITY CLOAK

Sometimes I feel like I've achieved that cool dream of going back in time to enter the world as an unseen observer. Except the time is now and I guess I have forgotten my future real life? It's a commonplace that women of a certain age become invisible.

So we might as well make the most of this new-found superpower. Things to do:

Take drugs over the border. Nobody would suspect you in a million years. Even though you look nothing like your passport photo, the border guard will glance through you and it and register the same daguerreotype of an ancestor born before the invention of the bicycle. That skunky pong in your car is probably just the way Death's breath smells. 'Have a good trip,' the guard mumbles, without irony.

Steal art. Two young men in coveralls feigning workaday purpose as they unlock the glass case will raise suspicion. But a menopausal woman? Dressed in vaguely curatorial garb? Perhaps a greige (dead snail) sweater dress and over-large necklace made of hammered copper plates stitched together with vegan cork leather? She can lift Janine Antoni's *Lick and Lather* (1993). The *Lick* half would be best. She may need accomplices for that one, actually. Seven middle-aged women in dead-snail greige would be even more invisible than invisible. As with black holes, you'd only know they were there because of how they affect their surroundings: the seven chocolate busts floating through the gallery, a wet eye hollowing out, bite-sized hunks of cheek and shoulder chipping off as they drift.

Sneak into a hotel room and trash it. Or even enter a hotel room legitimately and trash it. 'I don't recall anyone checking in to that room,' the young fellow at the front desk will protest. Cameras will be installed. But they pick up only chairs flying across the room, mirrors splintering, feathers erupting from slaloming pillows, champagne bottles bobbing in the air and then shooting foam everywhere. The recording might pick up some garbled cackling.

There's no such thing as poltergeists. All the phenomena ever attributed to them were hijinks performed by women over fifty. You just couldn't see them.

44. THOUGHTS OF MORTALITY

From her booster in the back seat Elise first notices the Ruthven graveyard. 'Can we go to the playground?'

'That's actually a cemetery.'

'What's a cementery?'

Okay. 'Well, when people die, we bury them in the ground and those stones tell us their names so we can remember them.'

The rear-view mirror frames a thoroughly aghast small face. I need to spin this. 'But, you know, it's really just their bodies that we put down there.'

Her eyes only widen further and she's almost afraid to ask, 'Where do they put ... the *heads*?!'

Where indeed.

In the seminar room where we hold our faculty meetings, four five-gallon wide-mouth jars of water loom from atop the highest bookcase. In them float printed transparencies of heads: W. O. Mitchell, Marshall McLuhan, Alistair MacLeod, and Joyce Carol Oates, luminaries who have taught in our department. (Joyce Carol Oates is not dead, but she has written more than one lifetime's worth of literature. Also she did move to the U.S.). On Bring Your Child to Work Day, Elise starts putting two and two together.

Brushes with the mystery of death begin in childhood and arise, depending on one's life experience, with variable frequency and brutality as the years pass. I do notice, though, that it's at my age when many people first realize they are *for real* going to die one day. This may have something to do with the transitions of menopause, but I think it's also a numbers trick. Fifty. Traditionally, when a man starts cruising around in the bottom half of a car and a woman palpates a perfectly ripe avocado in the fruit bowl and decides, rather than saving it for someone else until it shrivels, goes punky, and rolls into the compost, to eat it herself right then and there. Then they divorce. Fifty. Half-way there, though statistically speaking 100 is a long shot, so we are already well into the second half. I used to think it so sad my Grandpa, dying at seventy-six, missed out on the Fourth Quarter he wrote so much about, but in truth he almost finished out the game.

While historical literature often proposes that there's a link between menopause and death (or that there should be – cleric Thomas Becon, borrowing from Matthew, reasoned that trees no longer bearing fruit are 'hewen downe and cast into the fyre'), in fact women live many years beyond our reproductive chapter. Very few species do this, under ten that scientists are certain of. Guess what two of them are? Humans and narwhals! (See 23. Thinning Hair.) One of the billion Susans has written a book about this, *The Slow Moon Climbs*, where she lays out the grandmother hypothesis – in short, that homo sapiens' post-reproductive gals explain our success as a species. For hundreds of thousands of years, grandmothers have been driving kids to Montessori and fashioning Legos out of clay and tallow. Mattern's book explores the global and historical conceptualizations of menopause, and it is eloquent and super interesting, though some readers may start to feel that the discussions of cultural relativity conspire to suggest the sweat dripping from our ears onto its pages isn't real. If the terms available to me for a hot flash were choking and suffocation (as in contemporary Spain and Lebanon, or in historical medicine – consider Jean Astruc's 'étranglemans de gorge' in 1761), I would be totally down with that. I'm as much a constructivist as the next guy, but when Mattern admits at the end of *The Slow Moon Climbs* that she herself 'didn't notice any symptoms not attributable to something else' I have to say *hmmmm*.

Would I *want* to live forever? Would spanakopita taste as great if I made it in an eternity × infinity inches pan rather than a 9 × 13? How many indigo buntings do I need to see? (A lot, but …) Would that mean Putin is also president forever? (Writing this in 2024: please tell me that last question dates this book.) The only time I wish for immortality is when I walk into a library or bookstore and realize I will not have time to read everything. I still haven't read *The Bulking and Foaming Filamentous Bacteria of Activated Sludge* or *Anna Karenina*. And they keep coming. If authors would just stop churning stuff out I could make some headway. No more writing books allowed![6]

---

6. Except books about menopause. The working title of this one was a darling I had to kill. In 2006, Nora Ephron breached a taboo with her bestselling menopause book, *I Feel Bad About My Neck*. Five years later, Shari Graydon published a feminist response, an anthology of essays entitled *I Feel Great About My Hands*. I wanted to complete the trilogy with *I Feel Hands About My Neck*.

45. FEWER SHITS

I don't mean constipation; I mean giving fewer fucks (not as in lowered libido – as in not giving a damn, a fig, two hoots, or a rat's ass). I give not only fewer shits but fewer of the rats' asses they came from.

I used to give so many hoots about so many figs' fucks.

Roughly chronological: a sour milk miasma wafting out of my kindergarten cubby, Kirsten scrunching her nose and requesting cubby reassignment; failing at bubble letters; failing worse at baseball; having no need of a bra, getting nicknamed Susan Bosom; inability to do a cartwheel; whether I overshared at the party; not snaring the high school English award (Congratulations, Jane!); webbed toes; the lint on my tank top illuminated by blacklights in the lesbian bar, making me the 'before' Head & Shoulders man; who didn't like my poems; students seeing me in a onesie at the 7-Eleven.

I used to worry that my torso was too short relative to my legs. Did I internalize misogyny? Instead of serving the patriarchy by frittering away my feminine mojo on self-scrutiny, should I have celebrated my advantage in 100-metre hurdles? Probably nobody else noticed my odd proportions, right? But they did. It didn't help that *ten years* after I had Mrs. Elliott for fourth-grade Phys. Ed., she spotted me at an Orange Julius and declared 'Oh, it's Susan Holbart! With the really long legs and crazy short torso!'

As my legs grew throughout elementary school, my mother kept adding material to my pant hems, widening the rings as she went to jibe with the bell-bottom style of the era. I'd grow another inch, she'd sew another inch. My legs like rattlesnakes: long tubes with groovy segmented termini. This is one of those beautiful motherly acts I now so appreciate, remembering my mum at the sewing machine in the evening, fussing with the intransigent toughness of denim under that fifteen-watt bulb just so that nobody on the playground would ask me where the flood was. A confident kid could have pulled it off – swaggered Keds-forward in funky Wranglers accented with the blurred strips of a Rothko painting. But at ten I knew my segmented pants would just render me even more of a weirdo than I already was.

These days I will wear pyjama pants to the store, and while wearing them I will approach a stranger whose husband barkbarkbarks at her and tell her to lose him, and I won't tuck my piebald hands in my pockets, and I will ask my neighbour to stop burning electrical cords in his firepit, and I will write about peeing my pants (see 20. Urinary Incontinence).

This is the little stuff, of course. The 'What will people think of me's. As for diners gawking at me for eating early breakfast with a dudey-looking woman in a Waffle House; the intimations that I shouldn't raise a child; the assumption that as a pervert I must want to discuss, and engage in, sex with you, man I just met (see 16. Depression); the black pickup truck tailgating, then revroaring around me to display the rainbow-flag decal that matches my own except it is being peed on by Calvin – these micro-shits continue to bother me, but not because of shame. I don't give a hooting hill of beans what you think of me, other neighbour who gossips with me about the predatory nature of lesbians, or plumber who edifies me, in my own rapidly flooding basement, about how humans used to live for 800 years until homosexuals ruined everything. But you do remind me that there are fellow queers worldwide under constant and existential threat, that we have such a long way to go.

As for the little stuff, now I carry only a small mesh sack of shitty rats' asses for the week. If you frown at the socks (left one grey, right one yellow with doughnuts) visible below my too-short dungarees on a Friday, you might not get one.

One of the bizarre things about menopause is that you don't know it's happening when it's happening. Classic menopause. It's identified retroactively: after twelve months without a period, you can say you were in menopause but at that point menopause is technically over. When you last cursed your curse you didn't know it was your last chance to do that. It's like watching a meteor shower. You lay an old towel on the grass and stare up into the starling-speckled sky, waiting for the Perseids. Every few minutes someone says *Ooh!* and everyone else says *Where?*, and sometimes a crackling bright one cleaves the Milky Way right above you and everybody says *Oooooh!* Was that the last one you'll see? You don't know.

Because it takes a while to write a book, I composed some of these chapters in perimenopause, some in menopause, and some in postmenopause. You have fully witnessed my Change. To honour the whole adventure I won't alter what I expressed in the pieces I wrote first, but to be honest sometimes I hardly recognize myself in them. If I saw the man in 6. Chills today, I wouldn't give a flying squirrel's left nut.

Gather your bad towel up off the grass and hike back home. There's ice cream there. Begin with strawberry.

NOTES

EPIGRAPHS. 'When describing': Foxcroft, Louise. *Hot Flushes, Cold Science: A History of the Modern Menopause.* (London: Granta, 2009). xx.

'And they're like': Gadsby, Hannah. 'Hormone Therapy.' *The Current.* CBC. May 15, 2023. Radio.

PREHEAT. 'involuntary laughter' ('des rire involontaires'): Astruc, Jean. *Traité des maladies des femmes.* (Paris: Cavelier, 1761). V.2. 309.

5. MOOD SWINGS™. 'uterus to continue': Aretaeus. *The Extant Works of Aretaeus, the Cappadocian.* Trans. Francis Adams. (London: Sydenham Society, 1856).

23. THINNING HAIR. 'You should be': Shakespeare, William. *Macbeth.* Eds. Barbara Mowat and Paul Werstine. (New York: Simon & Schuster, 2003). 1.3.45–47.

25. FATIGUE. 'Edison, who in truth': Derickson, Alan. *Dangerously Sleepy: Overworked Americans and the Cult of Manly Wakefulness.* (Philadelphia: University of Pennsylvania Press, 2014). 9.

28. SWARMING OF ENTRAILS. 'Swarming of Entrails' ('des grouillemens d'entrailles'): Astruc 1761. 309.

Satan lodging: Tilt, E.J. *The Change of Life in Health and Disease. A Practical Treatise on the Nervous and Other Affections Incidental to Women at the Decline of Life.* (London: John Churchill, 1857). Cited in Foxcroft, 129.

'Regurgitation': Astruc, Jean. *A Treatise on all the Diseases Incident to Women*, Translated from a Manuscript Copy of the Author's Lectures read at Paris, 1740. By J. R-n, M.D. (London: T. Cooper, 1743). 67.

'intense sexual ardour': Currier, Andrew. *The Menopause: A Consideration of the Phenomena Which Occur to Women at the Close of the Child-Bearing Period.* (New York: Appleton & Co., 1897). 194. Quoted in Mattern, 283.

29. DRY EYES. 'De Secretis Mulierum': *Women's Secrets: A Translation of Pseudo-Albertus Magnus's De Secretis Mulierum with Commentary.* Trans. Helan Rodnite Lemay. (Albany, SUNY Press, 1992). 131.

33. REDUCED LIBIDO. 'sexual neuters': Wilson, Robert A. *Feminine Forever.* (New York: M. Evans & Co., 1966). 25.

'fureur utérine': de Gardanne, Charles Pierre Louis. *Avis aux femmes qui entrant dans l'age critique.* (Paris: Imprimerie de J. Moronval, 1816). 405. Internet Archive. 10 October, 2023.

'Doing What Comes': Holbrook, Leslie. *Improving With Age: How to Enjoy Your Senior Years.* (Toronto: Deneau, 1984). 68.

34. WEIGHT GAIN. 'fat now takes': Corfe, George. *Man and His Many Changes or, Seven Times Seven* (London: Haulston and Wright, 1849). 73. Quoted in Foxcroft, 115.

'form becomes': 'Women in her Psychological Relations.' *Journal of Psychological Medicine and Mental Pathology* 4 (1851). 35. Quoted in Moscucci, Ornella. *The Science of Women: Gender and Gynecology in England 1800–1929.* (Cambridge: Cambridge University Press, 1990). 35.

35. ITCHING. 'irreverence': Cover copy. *Candide: A Comic Operetta base on Voltaire's Satire.* Composed by Leonard Bernstein, lyrics by Lillian Hellman. (LLC, 2012).

'bristles with': Propst, Andy. '50 Best Plays of All Time: Comedies, Tragedies and Dramas Ranked.' *Time Out New York.* 11 March 2020.

39. ANXIETY. *The Familiar Brown Jug-worm*: Calvert, J. F., and Cameron, J. H. *Zoology for High Schools.* (Toronto: The Educational Book Company Ltd., 1930). 39.

40. DIFFICULTY CONCENTRATING. 'any troll': Von Patten, Denise. 'Troll Doll History and Collecting Information.' *The Spruce*

Crafts, November 2019, https://www.thesprucecrafts.com/troll-dolls-overview-774728.

41. INDIVIDUATION. 'Sarah Yi-Mei Tsiang's anthology': Tsiang, Sarah Yi-Mei. *Desperately Seeking Susans.* (Oolichan, 2012).

44. THOUGHTS OF MORTALITY. 'hewen downe': Becon, Thomas. Extract from *Cathechisme* (1564). *Conduct Literature for Women, 1500–1640, Volume 2.* (London: Pickering & Chatto, 2000). 324.

'étranglemans de gorge': Astruc 1761. 309.

'didn't notice': Mattern, Susan P. *The Slow Moon Climbs: The Science, History, and Meaning of Menopause.* (Princeton, Princeton University Press, 2019). 369.

'Nora Ephron breached': Ephron, Nora. *I Feel Bad About My Neck, and Other Thoughts on Being a Woman.* (Knopf, 2006).

'Shari Graydon published': Graydon, Shari. *I Feel Great About My Hands, and Other Unexpected Joys of Aging* (Douglas & McIntyre, 2011).

ACKNOWLEDGEMENTS

Heartfelt thanks to my beloved friends and family who talked this project idea through with me, read, listened, and offered thoughts and edits that made the entrails of this book swarm more musically: Michelle Banks, Andrea Cumpston, Tom Dilworth, Alex Holbrook, Catherine Holbrook, Susan Holloway, Cindy Holmes, Nasser Hussain, Mark Johnston, Lori Kennedy, Nicole Markotić, Suzanne Matheson, Cristina Matteis, Jaksyn Peacock.

Special gratitude to Simina Banu, Elise Holbrook, and Ryan McLaughlin, wonderful artists and editors who also offered invaluable tech/design support, helping to realize the more concrete chapters in here.

Diana Luft, I so appreciate your generosity in helping me untangle the women's secrets of Albertus Magnus!

Thanks to Darby Bradford, who suggested that in subverting the parking lot man's gaze I took his power. Thank you, Maya Jessop, for inspiring 31. Metallic Taste in the Mouth.

I am grateful for an evening at my parents' cabin in August 2024, when my mother, daughter, sisters, and niece remained gathered around the dinner table and took turns reading chapters aloud. You made me feel I'd done something good for the gals.

This book wouldn't be complete yet if I hadn't received a Fleck Fellowship from the Banff Centre in April 2024. I got a room of my own in the forest and the inspiring counsel and good company of friends old and new: Derek Beaulieu, Silke Eberhard, and Meredith Talusan.

Elspeth McKay, thank you for so exquisitely painting the fan, easily my favourite part of the book.

And to the geniuses at Coach House! Thank you, James Lindsay and Sasha Tate-Howarth, for always cheerful and generous promotion support, Crystal Sikma for visionary design, and Alana Wilcox, queen of the narwhals, who propelled this book from the start.

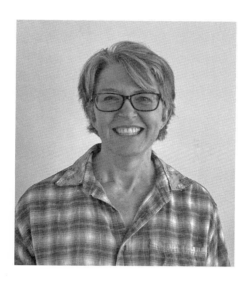

Susan Holbrook's poetry books are *ink earl* (Coach House 2021), *Throaty Wipes* (Coach House, 2016), *Joy Is So Exhausting* (Coach House, 2009), and *misled* (Red Deer, 1999). Her most recent publication is *Canon* (Zed, 2022), a chapbook featuring great works of literature translated through a calculator. She has also written a textbook, *How to Read (and Write About) Poetry* (Broadview Press, 2021), and edited *Intertidal: The Collected Earlier Poems of Daphne Marlatt* (Talonbooks) and *The Letters of Gertrude Stein and Virgil Thomson: Composition as Conversation* (Oxford University Press). Her work has been nominated for numerous awards, including the Governor General's Literary Award, the Trillium Book Award, the Trillium Award for Poetry, and the Pat Lowther Award. She teaches Literature and Creative Writing at the University of Windsor. She lives in Leamington, Ontario.

Typeset in Warnock Pro, DIN Next Pro, Leander Script Pro, Aragon Sans, Bright Lights Bold, and Courier Prime.

Printed at the Coach House on bpNichol Lane in Toronto, Ontario, on FSC-certified Sustana recycled paper, which was manufactured in Saint-Jérôme, Quebec. This book was printed with vegetable-based ink on a 1973 Heidelberg KORD offset litho press. Its pages were folded on a Baumfolder, gathered by hand, bound on a Sulby Auto-Minabinda, and trimmed on a Polar single-knife cutter.

Coach House is located in Toronto, which is on the traditional territory of many nations, including the Mississaugas of the Credit, the Anishnabeg, the Chippewa, the Haudenosaunee, and the Wendat peoples, and is now home to many diverse First Nations, Inuit, and Métis peoples. We acknowledge that Toronto is covered by Treaty 13 with the Mississaugas of the Credit. We are grateful to live and work on this land.

Edited by Alana Wilcox
Cover design by Ingrid Paulson
Interior design by Crystal Sikma
Author photo by Tracy Paterson
Fan, interior ants, and mice artwork by Elspeth McKay

Coach House Books
80 bpNichol Lane
Toronto ON M5S 3J4
Canada

mail@chbooks.com
www.chbooks.com